The Low-Calorie, High-Volume Diet

Make Each Calorie Count by Eating Nutrient-Dense Foods to Reach Your Goals

Bridget Blanton

is strongly recommended that you consult a physician, personal trainer, and nutritionist prior to commencing this or any other workout or diet plan. This guide is not a substitute for professional personal guidance from a qualified medical professional. If you feel pain or discomfort at any point during exercises contained herein, cease the activity immediately and seek medical guidance.

Table of Contents

Introduction

What's one of the main reasons why so many people who go on a diet fail? It's not for a lack of effort! It's because when you diet you have to eat less. So you really have to make the most of the food choices you're making. If not, you're going to find yourself miserable. Dreading each and every day with no end in sight and soon enough you're going to cave. Or you'll eat more than you should be and you won't end up making any progress. Either way is less than ideal, which is why we need a different solution. Something that will allow us to eat less calories but to where we don't feel like we're cutting calories at all. That's what my aim is to do for you in this book. I want you to be able to eat as low of calories as possible so you can lose weight in a way that's efficient, but also I don't want you to feel like you're even dieting in the first place. If we're able to achieve that, doesn't that sound like a pretty sweet deal? Well then let's not waste any more time and get right to it!

Chapter 1: Why Most People Who Go on a Low-Calorie Crash Diet Fail Miserably

I've already talked about this briefly in the intro, but why is it that so many people who go on a low-calorie diet end up failing? Even for the people who are able to see success, most are not successful in managing the weight after they've lost it. I think it's important to look at the factors that hold people back so we know what needs to be avoided when it comes to our dieting approach.

Too Big of a Gap

The first reason why most people fail is because the initial gap of calories that people are eating is too large. What I mean by this is the gap between what someone is eating before their diet and during their diet is too large. Yes, the goal is to create a good-sized deficit so that we lose weight at a good pace, but for most people, they bite off more than they can chew. Let's say for example someone is currently gaining weight at a slow pace and is eating 3,500 calories per day. They need to eat 2,400 to start losing weight at a good pace. That's a big-sized gap because they first have to eat less to break even and stop gaining weight, but then they have to eat below that to ensure that they can start losing weight. Jumping into a big caloric difference like this can certainly be hard for people to adjust to if they're not doing things properly. And that's typically what will happen, the calories are just too low compared to what they're used to eating. Once that initial motivation starts to wear off, it gets really hard to keep up with the low calories and so people end up quitting. Imagine if your income suddenly decreased by 30%. That would be challenging to adjust your spending habits to make up for the loss of income. Or to think of it in a different way if you wanted to increase your income by 30%, it probably isn't going to increase by 30% in one fell swoop. It's going to happen steadily over time until you eventually reach your goal. So to combat this we either have to be strategic so we can cut our calories in one fell swoop and not be affected by it, or we have to take a more steady approach to reach the low amount of calories that we're aiming to reach. Trying to do things in a more traditional manner is only going to lead us to a path to failure and that is evident by the lack of success that most people see when they go on a traditional diet.

I've Tried It Myself

When I was first trying to lose weight to get in shape, I went all out and I truly mean all out. I did everything I thought I needed to do to lose weight. And sure I did lose weight but my approach to doing so was terrible. For starters, I ate 6 meals a day. There's nothing good or bad with doing this (1), it really comes down to personal preference. However, I was cutting my calories so low that each meal was barely anything. How low was I cutting my calories? I was eating as little as 1,200 per day. This means that each meal I was eating only contained about 200 calories. I went around hungry all day. I would just wait for my next meal so that I could eat something and once I was done, I was still hungry. I would eat a pack of tuna sandwiched in between two dry pieces of bread with no condiments or anything. I would eat a can of unsalted beans for another meal. Everything I ate was super bland and dry. I never looked forward to anything that I was eating. Basically, each and every day was complete misery. Oh yeah and of course no junk food was allowed ever. I remember being around my family with them eating delicious barbecue and chocolate chip cookies for dessert and I was just staring at them wishing that I could indulge. Instead, I just sat there eating my catfish picking the breading off of it because that's how strict I was being. I just remember telling myself that it would all be worth it and to just keep pushing myself. And that's what I did. I continued to push myself harder and harder each and every day. And this isn't even to mention what I was doing for exercise. I would exercise 3 times per day most days. I did one in the morning, early afternoon, and evening. In the morning I would do a high-intensity bodyweight workout. Then in the afternoon, I would do strength training exercises, and in the evening I would do high-intensity cardio on a treadmill. And I did this rigorous schedule 7 days per week. Of course, some days I would only workout one time per day, but still it was intense. And can you guess what happened? On my third week of this extreme diet and exercise plan, I was doing one of my high-intensity bodyweight workouts and I blacked out for a second while I was doing some jump squats. I reluctantly cut the workout short and called it a day. However, this was the point of no return for me. Yes, I had gotten some pretty good results from this crazy plan which wasn't even that good, to be honest with you. But I realized that if I had to continue doing this to reach my goals and keep them, then it just wasn't worth it to me. I had to figure out a different way to go about things. And don't get me wrong, it was awesome that I was able to see noticeable results in a short timeframe. I liked that aspect of what I was doing. The problem was that it was just a bit too much. It was too extreme to the point where I was hungry, low on energy, and miserable all of the time. It truly felt like I was being owned by my fitness routine. I now understand that there needs to be more balance. You need to be the one who's in control of your fitness routine, not the other way around. You should feel like your diet plan isn't a burden to you, and your diet plan should be effective enough to where you're still able to achieve results quickly enough to where you stay motivated. Yes, that was the start of my fitness journey and it didn't go well, but I learned from it so that I could figure something else out, and now you can learn from it too.

Simply too Hard to Maintain

Another reason why going on a low-calorie diet can be so tough is because it's too hard to maintain. As I learned from my own experience, when you go extreme in the wrong way, you set yourself to crash and burn. Each person is different though. We all have different starting points, different levels of fitness and conditioning, and different things our bodies are used to. For instance, if you told a professional athlete to workout twice per day 7 days per week, they could probably handle it because their work volume would already be similar to that. If you took someone like myself who was just starting their journey at the time and told them to workout twice a day 7 days per week, their body simply isn't accustomed to that type of volume. So their body is going to breakdown and crash and they won't be able to handle it sooner than later. This is exactly what happened to me. I continually broke my muscles and my body down, but I never gave it a chance to rest and recover from the workload that I was doing. Eventually, things broke down to a point that I couldn't overcome and that's when I knew I needed to try something different. But if I had steadily built my way up to that, it likely would have gone better because

I would be giving my body a chance to adapt to what I was doing. This is what happens with athletes. It's not like they start out as professionals working out multiple times a day just about every day. Instead, they start out in a youth league where they might only practice a couple of times per week. Then it's on to junior varsity and varsity in high school where they're practicing for a couple of hours 5 days per week after school. Then it's college where the volume is higher than it was in high school and onto the pros where it's the athletes only focus, and by this point, their bodies are more accustomed to all of the exercise that the sport is going to demand of them. Another way to think about it is like a car. Imagine if you continually drove your car, and instead of stopping to get gas or get an oil change, you just continued to push your car to the limits and drive more. What's going to happen? You're going to run out of gas and eventually oil, and your car isn't going to run at all! I know that may sound like a silly example, but this is what I was doing. I wasn't stopping to fill up my car with gas even when I had the warning light on and eventually, my car, aka my body, just wouldn't run anymore! So one key to making a low-calorie diet work for you is understanding your starting point and understanding your limits. This will give you a good base to start from. And don't worry, this will be a big part of our dieting game plan. If I just give you some generic advice, you're bound to fail just like most everyone else. You're bound to push yourself beyond your limits and do things that you won't be able to keep up with. This is exactly what happened to me and it's why I was only able to last for 3 weeks. I didn't stop and think about where I was starting from and what my limits were. Taking some time to stop and plan this out like we're going to do is going to set us apart from everyone else out there who's trying to get in better shape.

Why Low-Carb Diets Fall Flat on Their Face

What's another reason why so many people fail miserably? It's because they try to go low-carb! Make no mistake, this diet plan is not a low-carb diet. Yes, there will be times when we're eating low-carb, but it will be vastly different than eating 5% or less of our total caloric intake from carbs every single day. What I'm talking about here is the more traditional low-carb approach that people take where they eat an extremely low amount of carbs or no carbs whatsoever. Going low-carb is one of the first things that people try when they want to lose weight. It's the most popular method of trying to lose weight today, but just because something is popular doesn't mean that it's effective. In fact, for most people, they're just going to be wasting their time with this. Why is that the case? Well stop and think about it for a second. There are 3 main macronutrients: carbs, protein, and fat. If you completely eliminate one of those macros you now only have 2 left that all of your food sources must come from. As you can imagine that's going to drastically reduce the different foods that you can eat. So your variety is going to be more limited than someone else who isn't cutting out carbs. It's this lack of variety that I believe gets to people over time. It makes it very challenging to keep up with. There are carbs every which way you turn. Time and time again you're going to have to say no, and I believe that over time this eventually causes people to give up on the diet. The other problem with low-carb is that it doesn't consider the fact that there are good carbs and bad carbs. Typical low-carb diets make no distinction though. They fail to recognize that there are simple carbs and complex carbs. Simple carbs are the things we need to eat less of like potato chips, candy, and white bread among other things.

Complex carbs are things like beans, oatmeal, brown rice, and sweet potatoes. I'm sure you can tell just from the list alone that there's an obvious difference in the quality of foods that I just listed out. Something like dark red kidney beans are far different from potato chips. However, with a low-carb diet, you're led to believe that even something like kidney beans are the problem. Let me ask you this, how many people do you know of have a weight issue because they ate too many dark red kidney beans? My guess is you don't know of anyone. It's far more likely someone has a problem because they ate too many simple carbs. Therefore, our focus needs to be focused on less simple and more complex carbs, not completely dropping them altogether. We can talk all we want about ketosis or how this is the most ideal way to go about things. First off I don't believe low carb is the most effective way to go about things, even if it was easy to do. But regardless it doesn't matter if it's the best way to lose weight because you're not going to be able to do it for a long period of time. Consider this thought experiment. I'm sure you know of people in your life who have gone on a low-carb diet. I want you to picture those people right now. Think about where they were when they started, think about how much weight they lost, but then also think about where they ended up. Were they able to keep the weight off? I'm sure the people you know are much like the people who I know. I sadly don't know of anyone who's gone on any variation of a low-carb diet and been able to keep the weight off. I've known many people who have tried a low-carb diet. I know people who have stayed on a low-carb diet for a good period of time and have even gotten some good results from it. However, one time I'd see them and they would be on a low-carb diet, and then months later when I'd see them at another social gathering, they'd be eating the foods with carbs like everyone else. And I think this is a perfect testament to how the low-carb diet goes for a lot of people. They start out good, you see them at a gathering and they're being selective about what they're eating. Everything seems to be going good, but you don't know the internal battle that's going on with them. The carbs usually win out because the next time you see them, they're eating just like everyone else. So at this point, we know we need something that will allow us to lose weight at a rate that will excite us and motivate us to continue moving forward. We don't want to move at a snail's pace, start to doubt things, and then quit. And honestly, a low-carb diet does check the box of being able to get results quickly. However, it fails to meet other criteria that we need in our diet plan which is going to be that the diet doesn't need to be miserable. Completely getting rid of 1 of the 3 macros isn't a good recipe for success. I don't care that low carb is supposedly best because ketosis is allegedly a better way to lose weight than an old-fashioned caloric deficit. You've eaten carbs your whole life more than likely so do you really think it's going to be that easy to suddenly stop eating carbs? It's not! For years and years, people ate carbs and never thought anything about it. Now low carb is more popular than it's ever been and yet the obesity epidemic is worse than it's ever been. Something just isn't adding up with this approach to things and we need to do something different if we want to achieve sustained success.

Chapter 2: Why Going Low-Calorie Makes Sense (If You Do It Right)

So far we've discussed what some of the dangers of going low-carb can be if you do things incorrectly. However, this diet plan is about going low-calorie in a way that can be effective. There are some benefits to going low calorie that you won't be able to achieve with some more traditional dieting methods:

A Low-Calorie Diet is the Closest You Can Get to Instant Gratification

We live in a world where we come to expect instant gratification. When we order something online, we expect to get it the next day or within two days. We don't want to wait a week for something we order to come in. When we're hungry, we can go to a fast food restaurant and get a hot meal within a very short period of time. We can get on social media and immediately start swiping through videos and different content. If something doesn't catch our attention within one second, it's onto the next one. We can date online and instantly be put in front of hundreds of people that we could potentially date right after we sign up. In the modern world, we really have gotten so spoiled by the ability to have just about anything we want right at our fingertips. This does create a problem though because things are much different when it comes to dieting. It's not as if you can start a diet and then two days later already see noticeable results in the mirror. Instead, the process is more delayed than that. It will often take weeks before you'll see noticeable results in the mirror. And for most diets, physically seeing results is the least of your worries. For some diets, you won't even see the weight on the scale go down. You'll just fluctuate your weight but you'll never really get anywhere. You might lose half a pound one week, but then the next you're up half a pound. With a lower calorie diet, we can solve both of these issues and most closely relate to the fast-paced instant gratification world that we live in today. When done correctly, you can lose weight in a way that motivates you and allows you to see noticeable progress faster than anything else you could do. Sure, no matter what you do, it will still take at least a few weeks for you to see noticeable changes, but nothing is more motivating than seeing changes in a mirror. This will start to create a positive feedback loop. Once you get some initial results, you'll be motivated to continue doing what you're doing even if it is a bit challenging at times. Then because your actions are on point, you will continue to get results, which will show up in the mirror, and this will continue to motivate you, and on and on it can go. Once this positive momentum is on your side, it can turn you into an unstoppable force. Be careful though as it doesn't take much to break this loop, and negative feedback loops are much easier to form and much harder to break. Sadly for most people, their diet isn't going to be set up in a way to allow this positive feedback loop to occur. Most diets set people up for a negative feedback loop to occur. You start the diet, don't see results, this discourages you, you become more reluctant to continue, you continue to not see results, and eventually you quit due to the lack of progress you're making. Luckily with this diet plan, that is not going to be an issue.

Keeps You Motivated When You See the Scale Change

Let's say you started a business. You want to become an influencer online and sell products via paid promotions. The first step to getting companies to reach out to you and give you products to promote is you have to have a big enough audience to promote to. To gain more of an audience you start posting. You make a post every single day, but the followers aren't coming. You're not too worried at this point because it's only been one week. After a month of making content, you're a little discouraged because you've only gained 6 new followers. Each of your posts are only getting a handful of likes and the results aren't what you thought they would be at this point considering the amount of effort that you had put in up to this point. You weren't thinking you'd be an influencer after just one month of posting, but you thought the results would be better than what they have been thus far. At this rate, you feel like you'll never reach your goal and soon enough you give up on it all together. In much the same way this is how we can think about weight loss. If someone has a lot of weight to lose, such as let's say 50+ pounds, then that goal is going to take a while to achieve, just like how it's going to take some time to build up a good-sized following on social media. Whether it's weight loss or building a following, everyone knows that it's not going to happen overnight, but we still have expectations for the type of progress that we should be making. If we've been posting for a month and have only gained 6 followers after posting every single day, that's not the type of results that you would expect to see. Just like if you've been following your diet properly and you've only lost half a pound after a month, you would be disappointed. Yes, half a pound is better than nothing, but it doesn't align with the amount of effort that you've been putting in. Imagine though if after your first month, you lost at least 5 pounds. Even if you have an ultimate goal of losing 50 pounds, 5 pounds in one month is a great start towards your goal and you'll reach your goal in less than a year, which is a really good pace. But do you see the difference? Do you see how in one scenario you're starting to get discouraged and after the first month you'll start to contemplate quitting if you haven't already? In the second scenario, you've done enough to lose a good amount of weight to encourage you to keep on moving forward. The trick is to make sure our approach is good so we can continue to maintain that pace.

Get to Maintenance Faster

Another important thing we have to think about in regards to how fast we want to lose weight is that the faster we reach our goal, the faster we can get to maintain calories. Why does that matter you ask? Well, think about it, when you're trying to lose weight, you have to consume less calories than you normally would. However, things will change when you're simply trying to maintain your current bodyweight. At this point, you'll be able to eat more so that you neither gain nor lose weight. So if you're creating a larger deficit of 750-1,000+ calories, then this means once you reach your goal, you get those calories back. You won't continue eating the same amount of calories that you were eating to lose weight in the first place. So let's say someone ate 750 less calories per day to lose weight. They'll reach their goal faster than someone who's eating 250 less calories per day, and once they reach their goal they now get to add those 750 calories back into their diet. If this hypothetical person was originally eating 2,200 calories per day, they would then start eating 1,450 calories per day to start losing weight. Then once the goal is hit they now get to go back up to around that 2,200 mark. Not only do you get to have the extra motivation that's going to come with losing weight at a quicker pace, but you'll be able to add those calories back in once you do reach your goal sooner, as opposed to someone who takes things at a slower pace.

You're Not Driving Through Fog

I want you to picture for a second what it's like to drive through heavy fog. And let's say you're driving in an area you're unfamiliar with. When you're driving through the fog you can barely see in front of you and you don't know what's next. You just have to trust in where you're going and what you're able to see that's right in front of you. It's obviously no fun to drive this way, but that's what it's like when you're on a diet plan that you're unsure about to begin with. And when the results are slow to roll in, you start to doubt where you're going. The only problem is that you don't know where to turn next because of the heavy fog. However, with this diet plan, that fog will be lifted. Think about what it's like driving normally. You can see well ahead of your car. You can see other cars in front of you, you can pass other cars, and everything becomes much easier. That's what things are going to be like for you on this diet plan. You'll be able to see far in advance so nothing is going to catch you off guard or make you doubt if you're going in the right direction. For most people, this is far from the case. Most diet plans are the equivalent of trying to drive in a thick heavy fog, and all that does is make things more challenging than they need to be.

Why You Need High-Volume Foods When You're Losing Weight

The main reason why this diet plan is going to be so effective is because we're going to incorporate high-volume foods into the plan. Think about this like getting more for less. You see, on the surface what would you say is a better value: Paying $30,000 for a new car that's your regular everyday car, or paying $80,000 for a luxury car? In terms of the value when comparing necessities to a luxury car, most people are going to say that the $30,000 car is a better value. Imagine though that your budget was really tight and you still chose to buy the $80,000 vehicle over the $30,000 vehicle. You don't need to be a financial expert to agree that choosing the luxury vehicle isn't a smart idea. It's going to put too much stress and strain on your budget and it will make it far more likely that you'll have to take on credit card debt to be able to pay for all of your normal expenses. Even if you do have a lot of money, there's always the opportunity cost when you indulge in something that's a luxury because that extra money you're spending on a premium product could be invested or spent on something else. Therefore, it always makes sense to be discerning with your financial purchases, and we can think of our diet in much the same way. When you go on a diet, you have a calorie budget similar to how you would have a budget for your finances. When you're trying to lose weight, your budget is going to be tighter than it usually is. This means you're going to have less room for luxuries, which in this case is going to be things like those tasty treats that we all know and love. However, it also means we're going to have less room for things that seem like a good value on the surface, but aren't in reality. Going back to the car example, if one dealership was selling a car for $30,000 and another dealership was selling the same car for $35,000, which dealership are you going to buy from? The answer is rather obvious, right? You're going to go where the best deal is. Sadly though when it comes to our diet, people often buy the $35,000 car over the $30,000 without even realizing it. You see, it's obvious to know you can't afford the $80,000 car, just like it's obvious to know you need to eat less junk food if you want to lose weight. That's not what I'm talking about here. Instead, it's like going and buying the same car at a dealership that's slightly overpriced and the price is close enough to where you don't really notice it like you would with the difference between a regular car and a luxury car. That's what gets a lot of people. The difference is small enough to where they don't notice. But the difference is there whether you see it or not, and it is going to hinder you. You're going to step on the scale and wonder why the number isn't budging. So what would be some examples of this? It could be something like thinking regular pasta is fine to eat so you consume white pasta over whole wheat. Or it could be that someone eats pizza which they know isn't healthy, but they cut back since they know they need to eat less and end up eating one slice instead of two so things fit within their calorie budget. At the surface level, neither of these things appear to be that bad. Especially for the person who's being conscious enough to eat one slice of pizza instead of 2. And yes, I am a proponent of doing things like that so you get an opportunity to enjoy foods that you normally can't when you're dieting, but the problem lies in how often or how severely you try to do something like that and it all boils down to the quality of the calories you're eating. It's a similar thing for the person eating white pasta instead of whole wheat. You can look at the nutrition label for both types of pasta and see that the calories are similar, so any reasonable person wouldn't think there's much of a difference. They like the taste of the white pasta more so that's the choice they go with. However, in both of these scenarios, the amount of calories the person is consuming isn't the problem. The problem more so has to do with the quality of those calories. You might see that a serving size of white pasta is roughly the same as whole wheat pasta, but there's still a big difference between the two. The white pasta is going to cause a great spike in blood sugar levels which will lead to the pasta being more rapidly digested. The big spike will also lead to a crash, which will leave you more likely to experience food cravings later on in the day. With the whole wheat pasta, yes the taste might not be what we are used to or we might not prefer the taste, but it will essentially do the opposite of what the white pasta is doing. It will cause a slower release of blood sugar, it will take longer to digest, and it won't lead to a crash later on. This means you will be more satisfied from the meal and stay fuller for longer from it. So you're getting far more mileage out of the calories from the whole wheat pasta as opposed to the white pasta. The same thing goes with the pizza example where the person ate one slice instead of two. Yes, it's a good idea to do this strategically to help make things more fun and enjoyable, but the tactic needs to be used sparingly. If you do it too often you will still fail. And once again, it all comes down to the quality of the calories because it does matter. Let's say that a slice of pizza contains 300 calories. Yes, the slice of pizza will help to curb hunger, but you can get more of a bang for your calorie buck from other food choices. And over time if you continually make choices like this you'll eventually find yourself in a situation where you're choosing between continuing to be hungry or eating more than you should. If this person normally eats two slices, how full do you think they'll get off of one slice? They probably won't feel satisfied and so they'll continue to eat more to get full, and this is where the problem can occur. But do you see how subtle these differences are? It's like buying a car for $5,000 more and when that $5,000 is spread out over the course of a 6-year loan, it makes it a lot less noticeable. Most people have probably eaten white bread and pasta most of their lives, and the typical person might say they don't notice any difference when they eat white pasta as opposed to whole wheat or whole grain. The difference is there whether you think you feel it or not. And this is why the person who's able to make the better choices with the calories they do have will win out in the long run. They won't be fighting hunger cravings on a regular basis. They will feel full after their meals instead of hungry. And this is exactly what you need when you're dieting.

The Problem With "If It Fits Your Macros"

As I'm sure you can probably guess, I'm not entirely a fan of "If it fits your macros" (iifym), or flexible dieting. Maybe you've heard of this plan and maybe you haven't. If you don't know what it entails, essentially you have a certain number of calories and macros that you need to hit each day. So as long as you hit those numbers then you will still reach your goals. And believe it or not, this is true. So long as you stick within certain caloric and macro parameters based on your current starting point, you will see success. Why then am I not a big proponent of this diet? After all, it seems pretty good if you're able to eat what you want and still lose weight. That's where the problem lies though, and it's for the same reasons that I just described in the previous section. People don't seem to understand balance when it comes to dieting. They only know never eating anything fun vs only trying to eat delicious foods. And when it comes to something like flexible dieting, people do tend to take things to an extreme level where they're eating whatever they want and they're trying to do so within certain parameters. This is where the problem comes in. If you're eating nothing but unhealthy foods or mostly unhealthy foods, then all you're doing is making things that much harder on yourself. Sure on paper it would seem as if everything works out. For example, if you could eat 1800 calories per day, and you're able to stick within that 1800 calories by eating nothing but donuts and potato chips, then you'll lose weight. And yes on paper this is true and it will work to help you lose weight so long as the numbers work out. But in practicality is it easy to stay under 1800 calories by eating only junk food like donuts and chips? That certainly is a difficult challenge. Junk food items like donuts and chips are going to contain a high amount of calories but the food volume is low. These food items are also going to spike your blood sugar levels, which will lead to food cravings within a short timeframe after you eat. So not only are you consuming more calories but those calories are going to make it more challenging for you throughout the rest of your day to stay within your calorie parameters. So what do you think ends up happening with most people who take this approach when they do if it fits your macros? They end up overeating in one way or another. It could be by accident where they aren't tracking things properly and they didn't realize they ate more calories than they did. Or it could be where they're eating more just because they're still hungry. Either way, taking this extreme approach with "If it fits your macros" isn't going to work, but this diet is portrayed in a way that makes people feel as if they can do this. Even if you do realize there needs to be a balance, this diet offers you no way of knowing how you can go about achieving that balance. You're left on your own to figure it out and that usually leads to disaster for most people. They're unable to figure out how to properly balance low-calorie, high-volume foods with foods that they enjoy. In the end, this just leads people to their own vices which means that people are going to overeat. What it boils down to with this diet is there needs to be a better structure in place so there are parameters that can be followed. Imagine it like driving. If there was no median, how much harder is it to stay in your own lane? It's harder than you think when there are a bunch of cars on the road. Isn't it a lot easier to drive when there's a white stripe down the middle of the road? It seems simple, but having this parameter in place keeps drivers in their lane and it becomes obvious when someone is driving too close to the center. With "If it fits your macros", there is no median and so people end up drifting towards the center of the road without even realizing it. That's why with this diet plan, my goal is to make sure that you have a median so that you know the boundaries you need to stay between.

Chapter 3: The Low-Calorie, High-Volume Diet

This is where the fun can truly begin. We are now going to start covering the things you need to know for this plan to be able to execute and start seeing some results in a way that is sustainable for you. It's important to know ahead of time that there are going to be some things that you're going to have to think about and calculate out. I wish I could do all of the thinking and calculating for you, but I simply can't as I don't know you're starting numbers. You are your own unique person, so for example certain foods that you struggle with someone else might not have a problem with. That's why it can be so hard to come up with generic advice when it comes to fitness because if I tell you to stop eating pizza, that might not even be an issue for you in the first place. You could give up eating pizza but then still not see the results that you want because you're still overconsuming on sweets. It might be sweets that you struggle with more. This is why I can give you the boundaries and the exercises you need to do, but ultimately there are some things that you're going to need to do on your part in order for this to be successful.

Create Your Food Lists

The first part of this diet plan is going to be creating our food lists. What you're going to do is stop and think about certain foods and place them into different categories. Here are the different categories:

Foods You Can't Live Without

As the name implies these are foods that you have to have as part of your diet. These aren't healthy foods that help you directly reach your goal, like vegetables for example. No, these are foods that you love so much that you'd almost consider quitting on your fitness goals just because you enjoy eating them that much. And that's the thing most people will give up foods that they can't live without in order to try and reach their goals. Just sitting there thinking about it, how likely do you think that is to occur? It's not very likely, I'll tell you that right now. This is why a lot of people fail. Instead of finding a balance with foods they can't live without, they literally try and live without them. Take me for instance, back in the day I read some advice that you shouldn't eat French fries because of the bad fats that they contain. I listened to this advice and gave up French fries for a couple of years after reading that advice. I didn't want to eat something that would affect my health as badly as French fries could and have them prevent me from achieving what I wanted to do fitness-wise. So I decided to give them up upon reading what I did about them. Whenever I was around other people, it was so hard to watch them get fries with their burger, but I had to stick with just my burger. I was so jealous watching my friends enjoy their fries and I just sat looking at them in envy. I also felt weird doing this rather than just eating the way everyone else was. I'm not the type of person who likes to draw attention to themselves. Then one day I came to a realization. Do I have to completely give up something that I love so much in order to reach my goals? If I was able to eat this delicious food in moderation how much would it really hurt? Could it actually help me more than hurt me because now I would be getting more satisfaction from my diet because I could eat something that I didn't want to live without? And so that's what I did. I ended up eating French fries but less frequently than I normally would. Instead of eating French fries three times per week on average before I gave them up completely, I cut down to one time per week. This worked out really well for me as I was able to satisfy my salty craving, but not do it so much in a way where it ruined my progress. I no longer felt like an outsider when I was in a situation where I was eating fast food with my friends. I also had something to look forward to instead of just more misery. And so for me, French fries are a food item that I would consider as something I can't live without. Obviously yes, we don't need French fries to survive, but I certainly do enjoy life more when I'm able to eat them as opposed to when I'm not. And so that's what this list is about. Name off the foods that you really can't or don't want to live without. Initially, all you're going to do is list out the foods. Later on, you can come back and refine the list and eliminate some of the foods that more appropriately belong on a different list or aren't needed on a list at all. The reason we want to refine our lists is because we want to be really strict with what's on them. The more items that are on a list, the less of each item that you'll get to consume. For example, if French fries were the only item on this particular list, then I could enjoy them in a larger quantity compared to if I had 5 items on this list. Initially, though, you don't want to hold yourself back. Just come up with a list of food items that aren't the best for you but you have a hard time imagining yourself living without them. It can be anything like pizza, ice cream, chocolate chip cookies, just to name a few more of the items on my list. Once all of your lists are complete we can then worry about which list a certain food item best belongs on or if it should be on a list altogether. And it's also okay if some food items end up being on multiple lists. You're not limited to putting pizza on just this list for example.

Foods You're Willing to Give Up Completely or For the Most Part

Up next we have a list that will be not so much fun to think about or make because we're going to be cutting out things. Yes, it is nice to think that we can eat whatever we want and still lose weight, but ultimately some sacrifices have to be made to make the process easier. Sure, it is true that there's no one thing that you have to give up to reach your goal, however, it makes it easier when there are certain foods you know you're not going to eat. This will allow you to focus more on getting to eat the foods that you actually enjoy the most. Think about it in regards to your finances. Most people don't have a budget with their finances. They just swipe away without much thought and due to this most people aren't in the best situations financially. This is a bad recipe to rack up credit card debt. In much the same way, most people don't give a second thought to how it is that they eat. They just eat whatever their heart desires in whatever amount they want and this ultimately results in them being in a surplus, much like financially being in debt. So if we want to be in control of how we eat, we need to be ruthless with what we want to eat and what we don't want to eat. In much the same way, if you go through a simple exercise with your income, you would give up things that aren't worth spending your money on and this would allow you to spend more on the things that you care about the most. That's what the point of this list is. It will allow you to get more out of the foods that you can't live without. But this list isn't about giving up foods like fruits and vegetables. It's about giving up junk food items that you really don't care for. What are some food items that you never crave or think much about? What's something that could be right in front of you and you would pass on it for something else without giving it a second thought? For me, a good example of this would be something like crackers. It doesn't really matter what type of cracker it is, I just don't really care for it as a snack or otherwise. Also, notice how the list says for the most part. I do think it's important to note that sometimes you're going to be in situations where you're going to eat the foods that are on the list because that's what you have available to you. I don't want you to feel like your entire diet is ruined if you eat something on this list, which is why I've included the part about for the most part. I recently went on vacation to Florida and on that trip, there were definitely some times where I needed a snack to eat and all that I had access to in that moment were peanut butter crackers. Rather than forgo eating, I just ate the crackers and it wasn't a big deal. What you don't want to happen though is to eat the crackers and feel guilty about it or feel as if a big setback just occurred. That's why this is a list of food items that you're fine without touching unless a specific situation calls for it.

Foods You're Going to Need to Cut Back On

The next list that you're going to create is a bit of an interesting one. These are going to be things that you know you need to cut back on. Another way that you could look at this list would be your danger foods. These are foods that you have a high likelihood of overeating if they're out in front of you. So if you know you're eating too many potato chips and potato chips are something you can easily overeat, then this is something you would want to include on your list. The thing about this list is that there is likely going to be some overlap with items on this list and the foods you can't live without list. That's totally okay and it's to be expected. For instance, ice cream might be something you find yourself eating too much of, and at the same time, it can also be a food item that you can't live without. If that's the case, ice cream would go on both lists. What essentially needs to happen for food items that are on both lists is you need to cut back on them but not get rid of them entirely. Chances are good that if you're overeating something like ice cream or chips, it's because you like eating those food items. It wouldn't make sense to get rid of them completely. However, continuing to eat food items on this list in large quantities will make it challenging to reach your goal much like someone who wants to do "If it fits your macros" and eat nothing but junk food. There doesn't need to be a specific amount that you're eating of a food item in order for it to make it on the list. Just think about the food items that you regularly eat and what are some of those foods that you know you consume a bit too much of. What are the foods you feel are holding you back the most from your fitness goals? It's important to note that drinks can be included on any of these lists as well. I'm not referring to things like water here, but drinks that contain calories because calories from beverages count just as much as calories from food. The problem with consuming your calories from beverages is that most of them often do nothing to help you feel full. A soda for instance will do less for you from a fullness perspective than a bag of chips will. This is why it's important to think about beverages as well that contain calories, such as juices, sodas, alcohol, or even coffee if you add creamer, milk, and or sugar to it. Considering that the aim of this diet is to get the best bang for our calorie buck, as you can imagine soft drinks are the complete opposite of what we're trying to go for here. However, this doesn't mean that we want to give up something like soda completely if it's something that we really enjoy. You can just put it on your list of foods that you can't live without and the details can be sorted out later. I know for myself personally, potato chips are something that I can overeat on easily. This is especially true when I'm hungry and I don't have anything else in my home that's quick and convenient for me to start eating. So I'll just open the bag of chips and tell myself that I'm only going to eat a couple of handfuls, but the chips taste so good that it's easy for me to continue going and going and going. Next thing you know, I've eaten way more chips than I originally intended to. There might be foods that cause you to do similar things to what I've just described. And if that's the case, don't worry as I will give you some tips on how you can overcome this. It's not as simple as writing down potato chips on a list and then like magic you're not going to eat as much of them. What happens with these foods is they're convenient for us to eat so we have to change some things up to ensure the habit doesn't continue to happen, and I'll expand more on this shortly. Once you have your lists created, you can move on to the next step, but before we do that, I want to share with you some more advice on how you can come up with your lists in the first place if you're struggling to do so.

Create a Good Diary

When you're thinking of foods to put on your lists, some of them will be obvious and jump straight to the front of your mind. Other food items won't be as obvious. You'll think of them later on. And when you do, it's no big deal as things can always be adjusted. That's why it's important to think of this list as ongoing and not something you do once and is done for good. But something else you can do that will help you along the way is to create a good diary. All you're going to do is list out the foods you're eating for your meals. So if you eat a standard breakfast, lunch, and dinner, you're going to write down what you ate for those meals. You can keep track of this in a spreadsheet or a note app on your phone. Then you can go back and review your lists and mark off food items if any of them belong on one of the lists. This allows you to see what you're eating in your day-to-day life and have it act as a constant reminder of what it is that you're eating on a regular basis. This is more helpful than you might think because let's be honest with ourselves, it's easy to forget what we eat. We think we have a good idea as to what we eat, but I know for myself, I have trouble remembering what I ate for lunch two days ago. And that's the first benefit that this exercise is going to do for you. It's going to help remind you of what you're eating so you don't have to try and remember. This is going to make it far easier to complete your lists rather than having to do it based on pure memory. This isn't the only benefit that you're going to experience from doing this exercise. By keeping a food log, you'll now become more aware of what's holding you back. You'll more easily see what foods you're overeating on. Again, it's easy to think that we don't eat as many potato chips or French fries as we do, but when you keep a log that evidence is right in front of you and it's hard to deny. This awareness is the first step in being able to make lasting changes. If we don't become aware, then it's easy to think that we're eating less of something than we actually are. Not only that, but by doing the simple act of writing down what you're eating, it will be more likely that you'll make better choices. The reason for this is you won't want to log that you're eating more junk food so it can help act as a deterrent. I know for myself this is the case. Whenever I'm tempted to eat a couple of cookies because I'm bored or I just want a quick snack, I'll sometimes either skip the snack or opt for something better because I don't want to log that I'm eating something unhealthy. This isn't always the case but it surprisingly works better than you might imagine because it causes you to think before you eat. The question now becomes how do you go about doing this and how long do you need to do it for? Well, the first important note is that at this stage you're not trying to change up the way that you're eating. You want to eat as you regularly would. If you eat 3 meals per day, then continue to eat 3 meals per day. If you eat cereal for breakfast and fast food for lunch and dinner, then go ahead and continue to eat in that pattern while you're collecting this data. As I mentioned earlier, you can use a note app on your phone or a spreadsheet to track your meals and you're only tracking what you're eating. As of right now, we want to keep things as simple as possible and we don't want to add in the extra step of having to track the amounts of the foods that we're eating. So if for breakfast you ate cereal and toast with a glass of orange juice, this is how I would record it:

8/7/24

Breakfast:

-Cereal
-2% Milk
-2 Slices of white bread
-Butter
-Orange juice

It really doesn't need to be any more complicated than that! Yes, doing this for each meal is an extra step that you're going to have to take. Most people aren't willing to do this type of thing as they'd just rather eat. I can totally understand that, but I promise that doing this exercise will pay off in multiple ways because you'll have such a better understanding and awareness of what you're eating, and you'll have an easier time creating your lists. Just for the sake of creating your lists, this is something that you should do for at least two weeks, but doing it for a month will be able to give you a good amount of data that you can go off of. Even once you feel as if you have a solid list of food items, this is a good exercise to continue doing as it will help to keep you aware of what you're eating and what you can improve upon.

How to Cut Back on Trigger Foods

Once you do have a list of food items that you feel good about, you're going to need to implement some strategies to ensure that you'll be able to successfully cut back on foods that are easy for you to overeat. Make no mistake about it, if you keep things as they are, then nothing will end up changing. You'll continue to overeat on the same foods time and time again. Saying that you'll have the willpower to cut back on these foods is not going to work. It's easy to say that, but it's hard to do when you're hungry and you just want something quick to eat. So what are some things that you can do to increase the chances that you're able to cut back on foods that are easy to overconsume? The first piece of advice that I have for you is to buy your food items in smaller quantities. I know that you typically pay more per ounce when you buy food this way, but the benefit you'll get from it will be well worth it. For example, you can buy chips in a normal large-size bag or you can buy them as a variety in smaller bagged sizes. Another example is ice cream. You can buy ice cream in a normal-sized container or you can buy 10 for instance in a smaller size. The reason why you'd want to do this is because it will increase the chances of you not overeating on these foods. Instead of opening the big bag of chips and eating until you're satisfied, you'd instead open a small bag and once it's out, you're done eating. Sure you can always grab another small bag, but you're going to have to stop eating and then open another bag before you start eating again. Compare this to just being able to continually eat from the same bag, and not only that, but the bag is big so it's not like you're easily going to run out of chips. The same thing can be said when eating from a big container of ice cream. If you have a habit of eating directly from the container, then it's easy to continue eating the ice cream. If you buy ice cream in smaller containers, then there's going to be a stopping point before you can pick it back up again and continue eating more ice cream. At the very least you could put the ice cream in a bowl and that can help to contain the overall amount that you eat. By controlling the size of the containers you're eating from, you can more effectively control the overall amount that you're eating. The other piece of advice I have for you is if you have a family. If you're living by yourself or with roommates, it can be easier to implement the first piece of advice. If you have a family, then executing on what I just mentioned can be harder. It might not be practical to buy smaller sizes for your family or your partner might not be on board with buying smaller sizes, because let's face it, certain flavors of ice cream, chips, and other such food items can only be bought in larger sized quantities. You could be in a situation where your partner only wants a larger-sized bag of chips for example because they want a certain flavor that's only available in a larger size. You could also have kids in which case from a monetary perspective, it may not be the most practical to buy in smaller quantities. It's also not practical to completely toss these trigger foods and have them out of the home so no temptation exists. If the people living with you still want to eat those tasty treats, then you're going to be fighting an uphill battle. So what can you do? While it may be a little inconvenient, what you can do is buy a lockbox that can be put in your fridge. You can have your partner have the key to it and you're only allowed access to it during certain times. You can use multiple lockboxes to where one can be stored in your fridge, one in your freezer, and one in your pantry so no matter what food item it is you're needing to cut back on, there will be restraints on it. This will work well because when you're hungry you won't be able to just grab the food item you want. You'll have to ask your partner for the key and this deterrent can be enough to cause you to look for something else. Getting a lockbox for certain food items may not be your style, and if that's the case, what I recommend you to do is buy a separate mini fridge or a separate fridge all tougher if you have room for it in your garage or something else along those lines. The extra fridge will be for your use only and you'll store all of your food items in it, and the rest of the family will use the other fridge for their items. On the surface, this may seem pointless; what good does a separate fridge do if you still have access to the other fridge? Well, you could put a lock on the other fridge, but that will only make things harder to access for the rest of your family. Even without a lock, having a separate fridge that you will go to will help to build a habit of not going to the other fridge. Soon enough you'll just go to your fridge to get the food items that you need and this is where you can be in more control of things in regards to the sizes that you're buying. The same can be done with a pantry where you could buy a separate stackable shelf that you could store elsewhere and keep your food items on. Keeping things separate as much as possible is going to be the best way for you to avoid temptation. The next to last tip I have for you is to fill up on other foods first. Sometimes you're going to be in situations where you could overeat your danger foods and there's no barrier between you and the delicious food that you crave. Maybe you're at a friend's cookout and they have a big plate of chocolate chip cookies, and there's plenty for everyone so it would be easy to over consume them. Well regardless of the scenario that you find yourself in, what you need to do is fill up on other foods first. Fill up on the more dense foods like your vegetables and proteins first. This will go a long way in getting you to feel full in the first place. Then you can fill in the rest of your meal with foods like chocolate chip cookies, chips, or whatever else it is that you find tempting. Naturally, you'll eat less of your danger foods because you won't be as hungry at this point. If you start with the tempting food, then the chances are way higher that you're going to eat more of that food than you should. I'll give you a real-life example of how I recently utilized this tip. I went and saw a movie with my friends the other week. When I go to the movies I want to enjoy myself with popcorn and a drink. However, I know that I have a tendency to overeat on the popcorn if I'm hungry, so what I did was I ate a meal before I went to the movies and that caused me to eat far less of the popcorn than I normally would have. By doing things this way I still got to enjoy my popcorn at the movies but I had a barrier set up prior to the movie to ensure that I wouldn't overeat. Had I not done this, I would have set myself up for failure. It's easy enough to tell yourself that you'll be able to refrain while you're at the movies. Once you're there though, it's much tougher to restrain yourself. When you're standing in the concession stand line and you can already smell that buttery popcorn, it just makes it all the more tempting to get a size bigger than you originally intended to.

Do a 30-Day Challenge

One of the last things I have for you to try is a
30-day challenge. This is something that I used
to do back in the day and it works surprisingly
well. You can use this as a tool to help you
manage your cravings. The main idea is to help
manage your cravings, we're not trying to get
rid of the food completely here. This is exactly
where a 30-day challenge can be beneficial. In
fact, this is exactly what I did to help manage
my ice cream craving. Every night after I ate
dinner I found myself craving mint chocolate
chip ice cream. Sometimes I would eat it out of
a bowl and the amount I ate was contained.
Other times I would eat straight from the
container and I found myself eating way more
of it than I needed to. Either way, I knew that
the ice cream was in control of me and I was
not in control of the ice cream, so I needed to
do something about it. So once I finished off
my container of ice cream, I didn't buy
anymore and instead, I started a 30-day
challenge where I wouldn't eat any ice cream.
The cool thing about 30 days is that there is an
end in sight and it feels manageable. Even if
you feel that 30 days is too long of a timeframe
for you to manage, you could trim down the
timeframe to 21 days and it would still be

effective. All you're going to do is give up the food item for that length of time, whether it's 30 or 21 days. Once you complete this, you'll notice that your cravings for that food will either be gone or severely diminished. I know for myself with the ice cream before the challenge it was hard for me to turn it down. Afterwards though, I felt like I had a take-it-or-leave-it relationship with ice cream. I found myself not desiring it after my dinner like I had before I started the challenge. With this challenge, if you're struggling with it, you can try implementing some of the advice I mentioned earlier if you're unable to completely get rid of the food item from your home. Getting rid of the food item during the challenge is the best way to go about things because it will help you to avoid temptation altogether. However, you may not be able to do that if you have family members who still want to eat ice cream for example. So this is where you'd still want to have your own separate fridge or food area if possible so that way you're not being tempted every time you open the fridge. The other thing you want to do with these challenges is you want to do it with only one food at a time. If you do it with multiple foods at the same time, all you're doing is making things more challenging on yourself and making it more likely that you're going to give up. Instead, imagine if on your first month you did this with something like French fries and then on your second month you did it with something different like donuts. Now two months into things you've been able to manage your cravings for two different food items rather than potentially failing at trying to do two food items at once.

Determine How Quickly You Will Lose Weight

Once we've taken a couple of weeks to create our lists, it's now time to run some calculations to determine how quickly it is that we're going to lose weight. Remember, the key here is that we want to lose weight at the maximum rate that we can reasonably manage, and that rate is going to vary from person to person. What we don't want to do is push ourselves too hard and crash and burn. It's much better to realize we're going a bit too fast and then slow down on our own accord, rather than to continually go fast and end up crashing. The first step we need to take in this process is to determine our baseline numbers. What I mean by this is how many calories are we burning off in a given day? To determine that rate for yourself, you can use the following formula (2):

For Males: (4.38 x weight in pounds) + (14.55 x height in inches) - (5.08 x age in years) + 260

For Females: (3.35 x weight in pounds) + (15.42 x height in inches) - (2.31 x age in years) + 43

The thing that I like about this formula is that it takes multiple factors into consideration to ultimately determine your metabolic rate. Yes, it can be a little bit of a nuisance to plug your numbers in and calculate this, but it's well worth it for the better accuracy. Yes, no formula is going to be perfect, but this is going to be as good as it gets due to all of the different factors that are coming into play. At the end of the day, your age, gender, height, and current bodyweight all play a factor in determining how many calories you burn off in a given day. Some formulas only take into consideration your bodyweight, and while that may be simple enough to calculate, we want better accuracy. Imagine if you get this step wrong, you could cause yourself to eat less than you should be, which isn't fun. The other possibility is you use a formula that overestimates the amount of calories you burn off per day and that causes you to not lose any weight at all even though you think you should. That is something you don't want to experience, so it's better to take the extra couple of minutes and just get things right in the first place. Once we have this number though, that is only the beginning. We need to further manipulate the number we calculated so we can determine how much weight we want to lose per week. As a baseline, there are about 3500 calories in one pound of fat (3). This means that if you want to lose about 4 pounds per month or one per week, you need to create a weekly deficit of 3,500 calories. This calculated out per day comes out to 500 calories per day. Now, there are some factors you'll need to consider to help you determine how fast you can lose weight. One of the big factors will depend on what your number from the formula was to begin with. For example, if you're a shorter female, your initial number is going to be a lot less when compared to someone who's a taller male. Therefore you're not going to have much room to eat less calories compared to someone who's naturally burning off more per day. If someone runs their numbers and gets 1600 per day as their baseline and someone else gets 2600, do you see how the second person has a lot more room to be able to create a larger deficit if they choose to do so? That's going to be the main factor in determining how quickly you can lose weight, but it's not the only thing that we want to consider. You also need to think about how much weight you're trying to lose. The reason for this is the more weight you have to lose, the faster of a rate you can lose it at. For example, let's compare someone who needs to lose 100 pounds to someone who needs to lose 10 pounds. Let's say that both of these individuals are males of the same height. The only difference is their body weight. The person who needs to lose 100 pounds will burn more calories per day compared to the person who only has 10 pounds to lose. This is because body weight has a caloric cost to it regardless if it's muscle or fat. Yes, muscle is more metabolically expensive than fat, but the more mass someone has, the more the body is going to have to work to maintain that system. Therefore, the person with more mass is going to burn more calories than someone who weighs less than them so long as other factors like height and gender are the same. What does this mean? It means that a person who weighs more can eat less and create a larger deficit, which will in turn lead to them losing weight at

a faster pace. The opposite holds true, meaning
that the closer you are to your goal bodyweight,
the slower the rate is you'll be able to lose
weight. This is because you are already closer
to what your metabolism will be at your ideal
bodyweight. Additionally, since you're already
burning less calories compared to someone
who had more weight to lose, you have less
calories that you could cut. This is similar to
how a shorter female will burn far less than a
taller male, and therefore the shorter female
won't have as much room to cut back on
calories. If you are close to your goal
bodyweight, then go ahead and pat yourself on
the back because you're already on the home
stretch. It may seem like it's an advantage to
have more weight to lose because you're
burning more calories, but regardless as you
start to lose weight your metabolism will
naturally slow down anyways. So essentially if
you do have more weight to lose, you're just
further behind than someone who is closer to
their ideal bodyweight. The good news is that
you can catch up to them more quickly because
you have more room to spare in terms of
calories. You can afford to cut more calories,
lose weight at a faster pace, and get closer to
your ideal bodyweight. This is of course if you
want to cut more calories, but you don't have

to. You can still go at a moderate pace if that's what you feel you can handle. But this is one of the reasons why it's so hard for the average person to lose weight. Your body and metabolism are used to eating a certain number of calories per day, and then all of a sudden, you're going to slash the number of calories that you're eating. It can be a big adjustment for your body to get used to, and for a lot of people, they're not able to handle it because their approach is not that good. Either way, in regards to determining your weight loss rate, consider your starting stats such as your height and gender, and also think about how much weight you have to lose. Then bear in mind that if you want to lose one pound per week, you're going to need to create a deficit of 500 calories per day. So if your calculation from the above formula came out 2,250, you would take that number and subtract 500 from it for a total of 1,750. Of course, this is where the fun comes in. You can lower that amount if you think you can tolerate a larger deficit. Every additional 250 calories that you cut will result in an additional half a pound of weight loss per week. You can start with what you feel you can most reasonably manage. Yes to start things off, this will be an educated guess as you won't know exactly what your body can handle.

The good news is that it's not a problem because you can always adjust things along the way. Maybe you get started and two days into things you realize that you're going at a pace that is too uncomfortable for you. That's no big deal as you can bump up your calories to something more manageable, but something that still allows you to lose weight at a good pace. Maybe you go good at losing weight at 2 pounds per week for 3 months, but then you start to feel a little worn out from it. Again no worries, as you can dial things back a bit. You could run into the opposite issue where you feel fine, but you're not losing weight quickly enough. You can cut your calories to a point where you start losing weight at a pace that you're satisfied with. The real question becomes should you start out fast or slow? Well, the answer to that question is really going to depend on the type of person that you are. Are you someone who can be patient and fine-tune things as you go along? Are you okay with things going slower in the beginning so that you can at least ensure you're eating as many calories as possible and still staying on pace to lose weight? Or are you someone who wants to see results quickly? You don't care what it is that you have to do to reach your goal, you want to get there and you want to get there now! If you're the first type of person that I described, it's going to be best for you to take the slower approach. One where you start off with a simple baseline such as one pound per week. You'll see how you feel and you'll consider if you can drop your calories lower or not. Even if you do feel good at the rate you're currently going at, it's not a bad idea to cut your calories a bit and see if you can handle the new change. If you're currently losing weight at a rate of 1 pound per week, you could try out something like 1.25 pounds per week and see how your body does with that. If you're unable to tolerate it, then you can go back down to one pound per week. If you don't feel that change much, then congratulations, you're now losing weight at a faster pace. You can continue to play this game of dieting limbo to see how low you can go with your calories at a pace that's comfortable for you. If you want to take the faster approach, then you'll want to think about your starting point like I mentioned earlier, and then pick the most amount of weight that you feel you can tolerate losing per week. Whatever your starting point is, you'll want to see if you can handle that. If you're unable to, then you'll want to add in 250 extra calories per day and see if that gets you to a point where you can manage the pace you're currently going. If not, then you'll want to continue to increase your caloric intake by increments of 250 per day until you reach a level you feel comfortable with. I recommend giving things at least a couple of days, but preferably a week before you bump things up. This way you'll truly be able to know that your current pace is something that you're unable to sustain. As an example, let's say you punch your numbers into the formula and it turns out that you burn 2,750 calories per day. You'd need to eat 2,250 calories per day to lose one pound per week. However, you want to drive in the fast lane and you feel as if you can tolerate 2 pounds of fat loss per week. So you would start off eating 1,750 calories per day. After your first week of doing this, you decide that this pace is a bit too much for you to handle, so that following week, you start to eat 2,000 calories per day. And now at this rate, you feel comfortable with where you're at, so you continue moving forward at the pace of losing 1.5 pounds per week.

How to Get the Most Density Out Of Every Calorie You Have

We have arrived at the fun part. We're now going to learn how we can make the most out of the calories that we do have available to us. And this is really what the name of the game is all about. If we're able to ultimately consume less calories but feel more full from it than someone else who's consuming more calories, then we are absolutely winning. So the following are going to be my top recommendations for some of the things that your diet should be comprised of:

Vegetables, Vegetables, Vegetables

Leafy green vegetables are amazing for a wide variety of reasons, but they are going to be a top staple as part of making this diet plan successful. There are many reasons for it. The first is that vegetables are packed with multiple vitamins, minerals, and nutrients. This is a big key in what we're trying to accomplish here, but the other key factor is that vegetables pack in all of these nutrients while barely containing any calories. In fact, eating a food like celery results in a net loss of calories. This is because it takes more energy for your body to digest the celery, than the celery actually contains in the first place, so it effectively has a negative amount of calories. But other vegetables, while they may not technically contain a negative amount of calories, they still contain so few that they're essentially negligible. Take for instance broccoli, which contains about 30 calories per cup. Can you imagine anything else being able to do much with just 30 calories? Imagine how little of an amount 30 calories from a pastry is? That's practically nothing! But you can imagine a cup of broccoli is definitely a good amount. And even if you're worried about the carb intake (which you shouldn't be), you still have nothing to fear there either because most vegetables contain a very low or essentially no net carbs. Essentially net carbs are determined by taking the total amount of carbohydrates that a food item contains and subtracting the amount of fiber that's contained within that food item. And vegetables contain a high amount of fiber which means that net carbs will be low. Fiber is going to be amazing for our digestive health and it's great for helping us feel full. It's no surprise that foods like simple carbs such as most cereals, white bread, etc. are low in fiber. Whereas foods such as whole grain bread and brown rice contain a higher amount of fiber. And it doesn't take a rocket scientist to know which food items are going to be better for us when we're dealing with a low amount of calories. Eating food high in fiber is going to be a key in this diet plan, and vegetables fit the bill perfectly. When it comes to vegetables, it can be anything that you enjoy. Yes, leafy green vegetables are going to be your best bet here, but you can focus on what you enjoy the most. You can eat as many vegetables as you like as part of your plan, but you have to be careful. Why is this the case? It's because vegetables can have a bland taste, especially in comparison to other foods that you could be eating. Due to this, people have a tendency to use dressings like ranch and other such seasonings to make them taste better. This is totally understandable as eating vegetables raw isn't the most appealing thing. However, this is where the trap lies. You may be doing yourself good by eating the vegetables, but you can hurt your progress if the dressing is overdone. Yes, dressing doesn't have to be something you completely get rid of, but you need to limit the amount of it that you use. You can do this by measuring out the amount you're going to use before you start eating the vegetables. For example, you could measure out a couple of tablespoons of ranch, Italian dressing, or whatever else it is you're going to use and then use that to eat your vegetables. This way you're getting to enjoy the dressing in a controlled manner. What happens with most people is they freely pour the dressing and this causes it to be overconsumed. The other thing you have to think about is how you cook the vegetables. Yes, vegetables will lose some of the key nutrients when you cook them as opposed to eating them raw. However, if you get bored of eating your vegetables raw or you hate the way they taste, then it does you no good to try and force yourself to eat them raw. Instead, you have to strike a balance where you can still enjoy them. This is what I had to do with broccoli. Yes, I know it's best to eat it raw, but it was hard for me to eat a decent amount of it in that state. The only way I found myself eating enough of it was when I would dip it in ranch. What I did was I started to steam my broccoli and this made it much easier for me to be able to consume. I found myself eating a lot more of it with ease and it all boiled down to how I was preparing it. So play around with how you prepare your vegetables, and pre-measure out your dressings to help you consume more vegetables without having to add in all of the extra calories that mitigate the benefits you're trying to gain.

Incorporate Plenty of Protein

Another staple that we have to include in our low-calorie, high-volume diet is going to be plenty of foods that are rich in protein. Eating adequate protein is a key staple to losing weight. In fact, I'm of the opinion that a lot of people fail in their dieting quest because they're not consuming enough protein in their diet. Yes, you read that right, people are experiencing dieting failure because of a lack of protein. You might think of protein as something that's needed for muscle growth, not fat loss, but it's a big staple for both. Lean sources of protein are some of the best value for your calories that you can get. Things like lean ground beef, chicken, and turkey are a few good examples. But even if you're a vegetarian, there are still plenty of other good food choices like Greek yogurt, cottage cheese, and fish. And even if you're a vegan, there's a surprising amount of foods that have more protein than you might think, such as nuts, beans, and oatmeal. And you always have some fallback options, such as a plant-based protein powder or regular whey protein, if you're not vegan. All of the options that I've just listed here are a few of the many choices that you have available to you. Think about consuming a meal consisting of something like salmon, brown rice, and some spinach, compared to eating a meal with lots of simple carbs like you would when you're consuming a fast food meal of a soda, burger, and fries. Imagine how many calories each meal contains and what each meal will do to keep you full. Not only will you consume more calories by eating the fast food meal, but you'll feel hungry sooner than you would with the other meal. One of the main things that makes a meal like I described above so effective has to do with the large portion of protein. What can be some of the things you have to look out for when it comes to protein? Well, just like how vegetables are good for you and can be made bad, a similar premise can apply to protein. For starters, the type of meat that you consume might not be lean. You could consume ground beef that contains a higher amount of fat, which means you're consuming more calories overall compared to eating lean ground beef. The other issue that comes into play is what you're eating the protein with. With a burger, for example, you could be eating it with cheese and mayonnaise, in which case the calories from those items can add up quickly. You might be eating your ground beef with some spaghetti, and the spaghetti is white noodles, not whole wheat or whole grain. You could be eating chicken lathered in BBQ sauce. Just like with vegetables, there are ways that you can overdo it and put yourself in danger of not making progress. A lot of these things are so second nature for us that we often don't even think about them. For example, how many of us eat something rich in protein by itself? Most of the time, this is not going to be the case. Maybe if you're eating Greek yogurt, cottage cheese, or something else along those lines. For the most part though, you're going to eat it with something else and this is where things can get dangerous. Most people aren't going to eat plain chicken by itself. Yes, a good choice would be to eat your chicken with something like rice or quinoa, but most aren't doing that. They might eat BBQ chicken, eat the chicken fried with gravy and a side of mac and cheese. If you're eating a burger, most people aren't eating it with lettuce for the bun. It's typically going to be on a white bun and possibly with some delicious, albeit unhealthy, sauces and toppings. And of course, we can't forget the sides as most people will be consuming their burger with a soft drink and fries. This is where protein can be dangerous. It's not with the protein itself a lot of times, although yes, something like lean ground beef is better than a greasy burger patty, it oftentimes has more to do with the sides you're eating and the sauces

and toppings you're using. If you're able to
avoid these pitfalls though, protein is
absolutely a staple for you to have a successful
high-volume diet while keeping your calories
low.

Complex Over Simple

When it comes to nutrition and more
specifically our carb intake, it's better to have
the majority of your carbs come from complex
carb sources and less from simple carb sources.
Believe it or not, our goal with this diet is not to
completely get rid of carbs. Instead what we're
trying to do is eat foods that give us the best
bang for our buck. And you have to think of it
like this, is eating too many sweet potatoes,
oatmeal, quinoa, and brown rice really the
problem? Has anyone gained a bunch of weight
because they ate too many of the food items
that I've listed here? No, it's not because of
foods like brown rice that people have a
problem with. It ends up being the simple
carbs that people really tend to struggle with.
Things like white bread and pasta, French fries,
potato chips, desserts, etc. These are foods I've
talked about thus far how they have a lot of
calories, but they don't provide you with a lot of
nutritional value. This makes it harder for you
to stick within your calorie parameters.

Unfortunately, though, you may have a hard time accepting complex carbs due to all of the hate that carbs have been getting in recent times. A point that I'll keep coming back to is the fact that most people who go on a diet fail and therefore we have to approach things in a different way. Carbs are your body's first source of energy and unless you're in ketosis, your body is going to use carbs for energy first. My guess is that you've spent most of your life not in ketosis, which would mean that your body is using carbs for energy. Now imagine that you all of a sudden try to transition from using carbs as your body's main source of energy to fat. And this is after your body has been used to using carbs for energy your whole life. As you can imagine it would be a tough transition, but some people are able to do it. Most are not able to do it though, and if the name of the game is energy balance not seeing how long you can stay in ketosis, then why give up carbs completely anyways? Instead, why not eat more of the kinds of carbs that aren't a problem and eat less of the carbs that are a problem? That's one aspect of this diet. You're not going to abandon carbs completely. Instead, you're going to largely get rid of simple carbs and focus most of your carb intake on complex carbs. What exactly is the difference anyways between a simple carb and a complex carb? The bottom line is they're both carbs and they both serve the purpose of providing energy to the body so what makes them so different? It comes down to how your body digests them. There's more to a complex carb than there is to a simple carb, and it takes more from your body to be able to digest a complex carb. This is a good thing. The slower digestion time means that you will get a better bang for your buck. You'll get a slower but steady release of energy. What's the opposite of this with simple carbs? Well, simple carbs are going to be digested at a faster rate. This isn't always a bad thing as it can provide you a quick source of energy. This is commonly why long-distance athletes will rely on glucose packets during their races when they'll need a quick source of energy. Or if you feel that your blood sugar is low, eating some simple carbs can help you feel normal faster than a complex carb can. On a general meal-by-meal basis though, complex carbs are going to be your friend. With a quicker digestion rate, guess what's going to happen? The food is going to be digested and then you'll be left with nothing but hunger. Does that sound like what we're aiming for with this nutrition plan? Hardly! This is why we need to consume more complex carbs or

consume variations of meals that normally
would contain a good amount of simple carbs.
Here are some different carb examples that
would be a good inclusion:

-Beans
-Oatmeal
-Brown Rice
-Sweet Potatoes
-Quinoa
-Almond/Oat Milk over regular milk
-Lettuce Wrap/Whole Wheat Buns and
Tortillas over White bread
-Zucchini pasta or whole wheat pasta over
white pasta
-Plenty of vegetables
-Plenty of fruit

Wait hold on a second, fruit made it on the list?
Isn't that not so good for you because it
contains a decent amount of sugar? Yes, fruit
does contain fructose, however, the fructose in
fruit is much different from what you'll find in
processed foods. Here's my argument with
fruit; it's natural and comes from the earth. It's
not some processed man-made food item that
was comprised in a laboratory somewhere.
Again just think about it, how many people do

you think have a problem with their weight because they ate too much fruit? The problem for most people is going to be an overconsumption of simple carbs and bad fats. Fruit contains soluble fiber which can help to improve gut health (4) and it's packed with vitamins and nutrients. It also tastes delicious, so it would be a shame to completely get rid of it because it contains sugar. Think about the premise of getting rid of fruit because it contains sugar. If you wanted to eliminate fruit for this reason, then it would follow that you'd also need to get rid of other foods that would otherwise be considered good for you but aren't because they contain sugar. This would include things like sweet potatoes and carrots. Most people would not say that these foods are causing the obesity epidemic and I would have to agree with that line of thinking. Yes, most foods that contain a decent or high amount of sugar aren't considered to be good for us. However, how successful do you think you would be if you would cut out sugar completely from your diet? As you can guess, people who try to do this aren't very successful. The reason being is simple, so many of the foods around us have sugar and it's hard to go with no sugar for the rest of our lives. This is why most people don't last long on zero sugar or they'll eat things that they don't realize contain sugar in the first place. Even with foods that contain a lot of sugar like pastries, donuts, cake, and the like, you don't want to completely get rid of these foods. Scenarios are going to come up where you're going to want to eat some birthday cake, so why give it up completely and think that it's going to work? Instead, you can enjoy foods like birthday cake from time to time and make fruit a regular part of your diet.

Eat a Moderate Fat Intake

Yes, fat is important and it's not bad just like complex carbs aren't bad. Most types of fats are good for you such as mono and polyunsaturated fat. The idea that saturated fats which were once believed to cause cardiovascular disease is now being called into question by recent research (5). It's really the trans fats that you want to limit your consumption of as these can lead to health problems (6). Aside from that though, fat needs to be a regular part of your diet. On this low-calorie, high-volume diet plan, we're going to want to eat a moderate amount of fat. It will consist of the lowest overall percentage of a macro that you're going to consume. It's not that there's anything bad with fat, it more so has to do with the overall amount of calories.

You see, fat contains 9 calories per gram, whereas protein and carbs only contain 4 calories per gram. Really, stop and think about that for a second. You're getting the same volume but over twice the amount of calories. I want you to picture a tablespoon of olive oil. Think about how small one tablespoon is, but do you know how many calories are in one tablespoon of olive oil? It's 120. That's right, 120 calories from one tablespoon. I'm not saying these calories are bad for you because they're not. Olive oil is a healthy type of fat. Compare that though to 120 calories worth of brown rice. The volume from the brown rice is going to be far more. Consuming a moderate amount of fat has less to do with fat itself and more to do with being able to get more mileage out of the other two macros. What are some fats that would be a good idea to include as part of our diet plan? Any of the following are good choices:

-Olive oil and coconut oil
-Any type of nut
-Natural peanut butter or almond butter
-Flax and chia seeds
-Avocado
-Fish
-Eggs

-Cottage cheese

Last But Not Least, Drink Plenty of Water

One of the last key components of this diet is to ensure that you're drinking plenty of water. Water is important for many things in the body, and it can act as a powerful aid to help you lose weight. Water helps to lubricate your joints, flush out toxins, and help get nutrients to your cells. Since this diet is all about getting the most nutrients we can, doesn't it make sense to consume an adequate amount of water? What's even better is that there is research to show that drinking water before a meal can help to reduce appetite (7). The study was completed with non-obese individuals, but regardless of where your starting point is, I think it's worth giving a try and seeing how it works for you. Just try drinking 8 ounces of water 15-20 minutes before your meal and see if you notice any kind of difference. If you do, then great, continue doing it and have it as a tool in your back pocket. If you don't notice any difference, then you can disregard it. No matter though, water is a very important key to your success in losing weight. Most people don't think too much about ensuring that they're going to get enough water. They just go through the day drinking when they're thirsty and a lot of the time people are drinking something other than water. People will regularly drink coffee, teas, sodas, energy drinks, alcohol, and other such drinks long before they'd start to drink water. The problem with these drinks I've listed here is that these drinks contain calories. And it's not like these calories are going to do much in terms of your volume. They're empty calories and there just isn't a ton of room for those kinds of things when you're trying to lose weight. Water simply hydrates you better than what I've listed here. Sure, you can make an argument about sports drinks because of electrolytes, but those sports drinks are going to contain calories. If you're an athlete, then this can make sense. For the average person though, you're going to be better off skipping past the sports drink and instead just sticking with your water. Instead of consuming those extra 150 calories from a sports drink, wouldn't it be better to actually consume those calories from something you're going to eat? I think that it sure would! The last thing to discuss about water is how much of it you should be drinking. Well, ideally you should consume about half of your bodyweight in ounces per day. If someone currently weighs 175 pounds, then they would need to drink roughly 87.5 ounces per day. This isn't something that you have to be spot on with every single day, it's more so to give you something to aim for. It can help serve as a reminder that you need to consume more water and help you strive to reach your daily mark. For most people, they want to drink enough water, but it often becomes something we forget about or are inconvenienced by. I know for myself I wanted to consistently drink more water throughout the day. I found myself falling short of the goal that I wanted to achieve. I'm the type of person who's not going to go out of my way to get water unless I'm really thirsty. What I did to overcome this was I bought a water bottle that I would carry around with me wherever I went. And magically, I started to consume more water throughout the day. And tracking your water intake is easy enough. If you have a 20-ounce water bottle for instance, and you know you need to consume 80 ounces of water per day, then you know you need to drink your water bottle 4 times over. This is the simplest way that I've found to go about things, and if you're currently not carrying a water bottle around with you, I recommend giving it a shot because I do believe that it will help make a difference.

How Much Protein, Fat, and Carbs Should We Be Consuming?

So far I've described that we need to be eating a good amount of protein, vegetables, complex carbs, and a moderate amount of fat. These things may very well sound good but definitions of moderate or "eating a lot of protein" are quite variable. So how do we put numbers to these things? If I tell you to eat a moderate amount of fat, that might mean 30% of your diet to you. To another person though, that might only mean 20%. This is why it's important to put numbers to what I've been talking about. It's important to know how much protein, carbs, and fat you should be eating so that you can stay within the parameters of this diet that will make you successful. Here are the ideal macro splits we want to aim for:

-Fat 25%
-Carbs 40%
-Protein: 35%

At first glance, something may seem very off here. Why would we be consuming 40% of our total calories from carbs? The first thing you have to remember is when I'm talking about carbs, I'm talking about complex carbs. This is very different from eating 40% of your total calories from simple carbs or even splitting the difference and eating 20% simple carbs and 20% complex carbs. The other reason carbs take up as large of a percentage as they do is because of the process of elimination. As I talked about earlier, one gram of fat contains over twice the amount of calories that a gram of protein or carb does. If you increased your fat intake from 25 to 35% for example, this would greatly increase the overall amount of calories you're consuming for the same amount of volume. Naturally, this might make sense, but then you'd surely think the excess should go to the protein right? Well, there's something called gluconeogenesis (8). Essentially there's only a certain amount of protein that your body needs. If there's an excess, the remaining amount will be converted into carbs. With this being the reality of how our bodies work, there's no point in eating an excessive amount of protein. You might as well just eat the carbs to begin with so long as they are from quality sources. And with this macro split, we are getting in enough protein to meet our needs, which in this case is going to be better satiety and maintaining muscle mass. The carbs are going to help sustain our energy levels, and the fat will help with hormone balance among other things. All together this combination will work together to create the optimal environment for you to lose weight and keep it off. At this point, you know how many calories you need to eat and you know the macro percentages you should eat. Therefore, you can now determine how many calories from fat, protein, and carbs that you should be eating. Here's how you can calculate that using 2,250 calories per day as an example:

-2,250x.35=787.5 calories from protein
-2,250x.4=900 calories from carbs
-2,250x.25=562.5 calories from fat

When looking at these numbers it can be easy to get overwhelmed quickly. Do I really have to eat exactly 562.5 calories from fat each and every day? The answer to that is a resounding no, as that would make things far too strenuous. Instead, you just want to use these numbers as a guide and try to get as close to them as you can. For example, if instead of eating 562.5 calories from fat for the day, maybe you ate 630. It's really not that big of a problem because you would have a very difficult time being spot-on with these numbers each and every day. If you ate 630 calories from fat one day, do you see how you're still within the ballpark of what the ideal number is? That's still going to be good enough to help move the needle in the right direction and that's what matters. Plus it's not like the additional calories you'd be consuming from fat in this case are going to come from bad food sources. If you overeat on a macro, but the food source is wholesome, then there's nothing to worry about. Things are set up the way they are because this is the most optimal way to go about things. Make no mistake though, things will still be in a good place so long as you're eating calories from good wholesome sources. What would be considered a wholesome food item vs something that isn't? It really comes down to ingredients. Imagine eating some raspberries. The only thing in raspberries is raspberries. Go and look at the nutrition label for a breakfast bar and you'll see a long list of ingredients. The raspberries would be a wholesome food item and the breakfast bar wouldn't. In this diet plan, the more wholesome foods you're able to consume, the better off you'll be. Wholesome foods embody everything that we want to achieve with this diet plan. They have nutrients, they have fiber, they're lower in calories, they don't spike your blood sugar, and a whole host of other things.

They truly make your life easier, whereas things like simple carbs are far more likely to put you in a compromising position of achieving your end result. However, if you'll recall from earlier, we don't want to completely write off simple carbs, but we need to have barriers in place to ensure that we stay within certain boundaries. If not, it becomes too easy to overeat the simple carbs and it will completely ruin the diet plan. Be cautious though, it's easy to think therefore that the best plan of action is to never eat simple carbs. This is a fallacy as well. The success rate of giving up all carbs completely is very low. Yes, it would be nice to think that you're different and you can go the rest of your life without simple carbs, but why do that? Wouldn't life be more fun if you could eat them, but you just did so in a way that's more balanced? That's what I want to teach you in the next section.

How to Eat Those Sweet, Sweet Treats and Still Stay on Track

How do you go about eating delectable treats, but do so in a way to where it doesn't mess up your overall plan? The first thing I want you to do is put a number to things. By placing a percentage of your calories that you're going to eat from junk food, you create a barrier that you can stay within. Imagine telling a kid to play outside and stay close to the house. That's going to mean a lot of different things to different kids. Instead, imagine a kid going into a backyard that has a fence. There's a parameter in place that the child can't go out of. As long as everything stays within the fence, then all is good. That's the effect that we're looking to create here. So what's the balance that we're ultimately trying to strike? If you can eat clean 90% of the time as I've described above, then the remaining amount of time you can eat how you want. Yes, 10% of your total calories is not a large number and that's by design. It's easy to get carried away when it comes to foods that we love and that's why a more strict parameter needs to be in place, hence the 10%. The bad news is yes it is only 10%, but the good news is that you can use that 10% however you want to. For example, let's say your allotted calories per day is 2,250 just to continue on with the example from earlier. 10% of that number is 225. This means 225 of your 2,250 calories can be for your enjoyment. Of course, when you break it down like this 225 calories per day isn't much. This is especially the case when you consider that calories from junk food add up quite fast. Luckily though, there is a solution to this problem and one that will still allow you to stay within your 10% budget. What you'll essentially need to do is save up your calories. So instead of thinking of things from the point of view of 225 calories per day in this example, you instead save them. This could be 500 calories every other day or 1,000 calories every 4th, for example. It could even mean 1,575 calories once per week. You can break it up however you like to. Maybe you do like the idea of having one small treat every single day. If so, you can totally approach things like that. Maybe you want to wait long enough to where you can treat yourself to a takeout meal. There are a lot of possibilities for how you can go about this. The only thing that really matters is that you stick within your calorie parameters. More than likely the foods you eat for your 10% allowance will come from carbs and fat. So all you have to do is make sure you're still staying within the realm of

40% of your total calories from carbs and 25% from fat, and you're still good to go. The magic of doing this is that it will always give you something to look forward to. That could be something small at the end of the day or you could have something bigger to look forward to every few days. It helps to change things up and keep things fresh. Sure, the most optimal way to go about things would be to skip this idea and eat clean 100% of the time. Implementing this small tactic will help to increase diet satisfaction and make the diet sticky. What I mean by that is you'll be more likely to stick to the plan and continue doing it for years and years to come.

Chapter 4: Adapt and Adjust as Needed to Fit the Plan to You!

In this chapter, I want to go a little more in-depth with how you can adapt your plan calorie-wise to ensure that you're going at the optimal pace for you. This is going to be a very important skill that you'll want to develop because whether we like it or not, things change and that's the case with our diet as well.

We're Human

We're all human here and what does that mean? It means that things change. Our emotions change, our stressors change, our jobs change, the people around us change. There aren't many things that I can think of in life that stay truly static. What does this mean from a dieting perspective? Most of the time when it comes to dieting, people approach it from a static point of view. This means if I need to eat 1,950 calories per day to lose weight, that's how many calories I'm going to eat each and every day. As I've just said though, things change. For one thing, our emotions and feelings change. One day you could eat 1,950 calories and feel great. The next day you might eat the same amount of calories and feel hungry. You might take a vacation and it would be silly to think that you should eat the same amount of calories you normally do when you're back home. I'm a big believer that one of the best parts of vacation is the food. I love finding some of the best restaurants I can when I go somewhere new because I want to try new things. I like to see if I like a burger better in this city or that city. If I continue to eat the same amount of calories that I normally do, then I'm not getting to fully experience a vacation like I want to. Not to mention, I'm going to be with other people, which makes it all the harder because they're going to enjoy themselves. Therefore, you have to come up with a way to adapt to the ebbs and flows of how you feel and when you're traveling or dealing with a special circumstance in your life. That's exactly what I'm going to teach you how to do in this chapter because your diet should not be static. You need to know how to adjust things when necessary so that you can continue to see improvement. Instead what happens to most people is they try to stay rigid. Then life will naturally bend them with travel, work, children, special events, etc. and they'll feel bad about it. All you have to do is plan ahead and you'll be golden.

How do you adjust for special circumstances?

If there's one thing we know, it's that things will happen. Some of these things will be expected and some of them will be unexpected. For example, you know you're going to be going on a vacation or not. If a close family member ends up in the hospital and you spend the night, that's unexpected and it will still change up the way that you approach your nutrition. I want to help prepare you to be able to adapt whether you're dealing with expected or unexpected events. Let's start off by talking about expected events. These events are much easier to deal with because you know they're going to happen. This is important because it gives you time to plan ahead. If you properly plan ahead, then you'll be able to enjoy yourself on your trip or whatever else it is you're doing and still stay on pace to reach your goal or not be worse off than you were before. And that's the first thing that you need to decide. Are you looking to stay on track with what's going on, or are you just looking to maintain? This is a big question that you'll want to answer because it will affect how many calories you can eat during your trip. For example, if you're eating

2,250 calories per day and are losing one pound per week, this means your maintenance calories are 2,750. This means you can eat that amount of calories and not gain weight. Sure you won't be losing any weight, but that's not the point when you have something coming up. The point is to enjoy yourself. By switching to eating maintenance calories for the event or for the trip, you've now instantly created more leeway for yourself to be able to eat more calories and enjoy yourself. The other option you have is to continue eating 2,250 calories per day on average so that you stay on track. Yes, this will give you less wiggle room for a scenario where you're likely going to want to eat more, but at least you continue at your current rate of progress. As you can see, there are pros and cons to each choice. I'll give you the different approaches and ultimately you can decide what's going to be best for you. Let's say you decide that you want to stay on track with your current weight loss pace. In this example, you calculated that you need to eat 2,250 calories per day to lose one pound per week and you want to maintain that rate of weight loss. The thing is you're about to take a 5-day vacation and you want to enjoy yourself. You're not going to be able to fully enjoy yourself while limiting your caloric intake, so what do you do? Well, you're going to have to make up for things in advance of the trip. By eating less calories leading up to the trip, this will then provide you with more leeway to be able to eat more calories during the trip. This is the key because most people assume they need to eat the same amount of calories every day, but you can vary it. For instance, 2,250 calories per day equals 15,750 calories per week. If you eat 1,750 calories one day and then 2,750 the next, guess what? That still keeps you on pace for maintaining your 15,750 calorie threshold. And that's exactly the premise we're looking to take advantage of here. The first step in doing this is determining how many days you're going to want to eat more than you usually do. In this example, that's going to be 5. The next step is to determine how many extra calories you want to eat. You may determine that you want to eat an additional 1,000 calories per day on this trip. This means you're going to need to make up for the extra 5,000 calories before the trip begins. What you don't want to do is make the mistake of saying you'll make up for the extra calories once you get back from the trip. You'll likely never make up for the calories and now you've gotten out of the swing of things on vacation, which makes it easy to continue eating like you did while you were away.

Therefore, the 5,000 calories have to be made up beforehand. Make no mistake, this is going to be a difficult feat to pull off. As it is, cutting your calories is no easy task, but now you're going to have to further cut them to make up for when you're eating more than you usually do. What's the best plan of action for this? Since you know when your vacation is, I recommend making up for those extra calories sooner rather than later. Think about it like this, if you try to make up for those calories only one week in advance, that's going to be hard to do. You're going to have to eat about 1,535 calories per day during that week when you normally would be eating 2,250 in this example. This is roughly an extra 700 calories on top of the 500-calorie deficit that you're already doing. This could be too big of an adjustment for the average person to handle. If you start the process sooner, then each day won't be as bad. If you have 21 days to prepare, 21 divided by 5,000 comes out to 238. You'd then subtract 238 from 2,250 to get 2,012. This means for the 3 weeks leading up to the vacation you would consume on average 2,012 calories per day. Doesn't that seem a lot easier to manage than waiting until the last week and only being able to eat 1,535 calories per day? Of course, you can manipulate the numbers however you want. Everything depends on how long you're going to eat more and how many extra calories you want to account for. From there, it all comes down to how far in advance you want to plan. The more time you give yourself, the less you'll have to cut back on each day. Yes, it's easy to procrastinate and think you can make up for it a few days before, but then it doesn't happen and now you're falling behind. This is why it is typically better to just halt your progress for a bit so that you can have more wiggle room with your calories during these unique time periods.

What if you just want to maintain your weight while on vacation?

Let's say you are looking to halt things for a little bit, how would you go about planning for an event like a vacation in this case? The first thing you need to determine is how quickly you're losing weight. Let's make things simple and continue to use the example from above. You calculate your maintenance calories to be 2,750 and are losing weight at one pound per week for a total of 2,250 calories per day. Since you're looking to just maintain your weight during these 5 days, this means you essentially have an extra 2,500 calories on the house.

Basically, however large of a deficit you're currently eating, take that number and multiply it by the number of days you're going to be splurging. So if you were currently losing 1.5 pounds per week and eating at a 750 daily calorie deficit, you would take 750 and multiply it by 5 since the trip is 5 days. This comes out to 3,750. This means you would have an extra 3,750 calories to eat during this week if you were currently losing weight at a rate of 1.5 pounds per week. In the case of losing one pound per week, you would take 500 and multiply that by 5 to account for each day of the trip for a total of 2,500. This means you would have that many additional calories to enjoy without having to make up for anything ahead of time. If you want to eat more than an additional 2,500 calories on the trip, then you would need to determine how many extra calories you want to eat. Let's say you do want to eat an extra 5,000 on the trip. This means you still need to make up for an additional 2,500 calories. Doing this is much easier than trying to make up for the full 5,000. With this, you could start an extra two weeks in advance from your trip. This means you'd only have to eat 250 less calories per day on the two weeks prior to the trip. Then once the trip comes, you now get to enjoy your extra calories. Once the trip is over, you would go back to eating the same amount of calories that you were before the trip. And presto, just like that you've managed to go on a trip, enjoy yourself, and not have it halt any of your progress.

What About Smaller Occasions?

You'll have other expected events aside from vacation where you'll be gone for multiple days. Maybe you're celebrating your birthday or something like that. This won't be a 5-day long thing but maybe you'll just want to eat to your heart's content for one meal or possibly one day. You can still follow the same guidelines as before. First, decide if you want to just maintain your weight or continue with your current pace. Then decide how many extra calories you want to eat for that meal or for that day. Then plan ahead so you can make up for those extra calories ahead of time and you'll be all set. Let's say you're going out to eat for your birthday dinner. During this dinner, you want to eat an additional 1,000 calories more than you usually do for the day. You decide you still want to stay on track as normal so you decide to eat 200 calories less for the 5 days before the dinner. Once again, you can change up the numbers however you like so long as you're accounting for the extra calories ahead of time. Sometimes though, the unexpected will happen. You'll suddenly find yourself in situations where you have little control of what's available for you to eat. How can you best handle yourself when the unexpected happens and life tries to knock you off course?

How to Stay on Track When Unexpected Life Events Happen

Life happens. This is true for everyone, but we don't know when it will happen. Unfortunately, there will be times when it will be extremely difficult to stay on track, and that's actually my first piece of advice when you're dealing with a life situation. I want you to take a deep breath and understand that it's okay. Yes, our health is very important, but there are going to be times in everyone's life when something else is going to require so much of your time and attention that it's not reasonable for you to maintain the pace you're going on. When this happens, don't feel bad when you have to ease up. Instead, focus on what needs to be focused on. You can always make up for any progress you've lost later on, but some things can't be replaced. This was the case for me when my mother-in-law was passing away. She was hospitalized due to low oxygen levels and ultimately ended up passing away about a week later due to pneumonia. I spent a lot of time in the hospital that week and the week after her passing was anything but normal too. During that time period, I accepted putting a pause on my current nutrition and fitness routine. I was certainly eating more take-out food and eating from the hospital cafeteria. Her friends and family supplied a lot of meals after her passing and when you're grieving, how can you say no to delicious home-baked cinnamon rolls and chocolate chip cookies? During that time, my focus was on family and processing my emotions. That's what mattered most, and so that's what I did. As the weeks passed by, I got back into the swing of things. I didn't try to overcompensate or anything like that. I just accepted that it would take a bit of time to get back to where I wanted to be. And I was completely okay with that. If you're dealing with a tough life event, then it's okay if you need to put things on pause. You can always make up for it later on. Other times though, you might be in a situation that's unexpected, but it isn't taking up a lot of physical, mental, and emotional attention. For example, I was recently coming back from a vacation, and the flight was delayed for 6 hours because of a flat tire. Yes, that's right, 6 hours because they had to drive the tire in from somewhere else and that person got stuck in traffic. It was a whole mess. As you can imagine, this threw a small wrench in my plans. I now had to eat what was available to me in the airport when I was originally planning to be home in time for my next meal. So what did I do? I did the best that I could with the snack choices I had available to me. And then when it came time to eat a meal, I decided that I would eat some pizza. Yes, this caused to me eat more than I normally would, but I just did the math. I calculated that I ate about 600 calories more than I normally would have had the flight not been delayed. So then for the following week, I just ate 100 calories less each day for the next 6 days to make up for it. And I think this illustrates the choice that you can make. You can either overeat and then eat at your regular pace. This will essentially mean that hitting your goal bodyweight will be delayed. For instance, you might have a goal of losing 20 pounds. So far you're down 10 pounds, but then life happens and you gained 3 pounds. Now you can just continue at the same pace you were before and it's just going to take longer than it originally would have to lose those 20 pounds because you had a setback. The other option you have is to make up for the calories afterwards so you don't skip a beat. I only recommend doing this if it's for something smaller, such as the case of my flight being delayed. Trying to make up for extra calories over a 2-week period, for example, is a lot to try and overcome. It's best in cases like my mother-in-law passing away, to just pick up the pieces when you can and start again from your normal routine. It's okay if reaching your goal is a little delayed because of an unexpected event. When you are dealing with scenarios like being on a long car ride, it is important to make the best choices you can. For instance, sometimes your only option might be to eat something at a gas station. Yes, your options are going to be limited but there are still better choices that you can make over others. You could choose a soda, or you could choose water. You could choose to snack on some candy, or you could choose something else like beef jerky, nuts, or a protein bar. Yes, having to eat from a gas station isn't the most ideal thing, but nobody is trying to say that it is. It's more so about making the most out of the situation that you find yourself in.

How to Know When to Slow Down and When to Speed Back Up

The last thing we need to talk about in this chapter is when to slow down and when to speed back up. Most people don't even think about how quickly they want to lose weight. They just try to go about things as quickly as they can. If that's not done properly, it can lead to you crashing and burning. Even for the people who do take the time to plan out how many calories they're going to eat and set a target for how quickly they'll lose weight, they typically stick with that pace. I'm not saying there's anything wrong with sticking with the same pace. Remember what I said at the beginning of this chapter, we are human. This means our emotions change, our feelings change, hormones change, jobs, and the people around us, it all changes. Why then can't our dieting pace change too? If our hunger levels change, one day we might be able to push ourselves more than another day where we're feeling extra hungry. Therefore, shouldn't our pace change up when we feel like it's needed? Yes, the majority of the time, things can stay the same. The point I'm trying to make is that it's okay to speed up or slow down based on how you're feeling. You can adapt your pace based on your hunger levels. Let's say for example, that on Tuesday you're feeling pretty good. You don't feel overly hungry. Your normal pace is a 750 daily calorie deficit. But today since you're feeling good, you're able to push yourself and create a 1,000 calorie deficit. Then on Saturday, you're feeling a bit more hungry than you usually do. Rather than just trying to fight through the hunger, which could potentially cause you to eat even more if you crash, you decide to slow down a bit and eat some additional calories that you otherwise wouldn't. The additional calories that you eat on Saturday can be balanced out by the fact that you ate less calories on Tuesday. It's not so much about creating the same caloric deficit day in and day out. You don't even have to think about things in terms of a weekly deficit either. As long as month to month, you're hitting your deficit goals, then you're good. So if you're feeling good on a Tuesday, you can create a larger than usual deficit. Then it might not be until two weeks later that you're feeling more hungry than usual so you decide to eat more calories. That's fine because it's all balancing out. If your goal is to lose 5 pounds per month, as long as you're staying on track to hit 5 pounds, then you're good. Maybe one month you fall short and only lose 4 pounds, you can always try for 6 the next month or even just celebrate the progress you did make because 4 is better than 0 and you can aim for 5 next month. When you zoom out and look at the graph that is your weight loss journey, it starts to give you perspective. What matters most is if the number is trending in the right direction over time. And this is where things can get a bit challenging. Let's say your goal is to lose on average 5 pounds per month, but one month you lose 8 pounds. This is truly an amazing month. But this is where some people fall into a trap. They then think that they should try to either maintain the pace or at least continue with their regular rate of 5 pounds per month. The second option is certainly better than the first, but both could hold you back. If your original goal is 5 pounds, you lose 8 and think you can do that pace instead, you're setting yourself up to fail. You've now just dramatically increased your weight loss rate, and when a month comes that you only lose 6 pounds, for instance, you're going to feel bad about yourself. Let's say you lose 8 and then go back to losing 5 per month. This is fine, but don't get down on yourself if you only lose 2 pounds in one of the following months. By normal standards, this would be seen as a mediocre month. However, when you average it in with the 8-pound month you have, it averages out to 5 pounds per month. So you're still staying on track with your regular rate. This is why you have to keep a zoomed-out perspective. You could lose 8 pounds in January and then only 2 in August. When September rolls around you could be feeling pretty bad about yourself because you only lost two pounds the month prior. Instead of getting down on yourself, look at when you started, which to make things easy let's say that was January. January through August is 8 months. If your goal is 5 pounds per month, then you would need to be in the realm of 40 pounds down overall. If you're within striking distance of that, then amazing, that's what you should be focused on. You should be less concerned with a bad day or a bad month where you didn't quite lose as much as you wanted. Yes, I get it, bad days can turn into bad weeks, which can lead to bad months. Next thing you know, a lot of time has passed and you haven't scratched the surface of hitting your target. What I've just described is a complete loss of momentum. What I've been talking about is different. Maybe over this 8-month period, you've had a cumulative total of 3 bad weeks spread out over that time period. Yes, these 3 weeks means your results aren't perfect, but we're all human and nobody, literally nobody, is perfect 100% of the time with their nutrition and fitness. What matters is overall you've had far more good weeks than you have bad, and this is why your overall results will still be stellar.

Chapter 5: Track Your Mood and Energy Levels

What's another aspect of health and fitness that people never seem to think about? People think about their nutrition and they think about their exercise routine, but what they don't think about is their mood and energy levels. As I discussed in the previous chapter, things change because we're human. Things aren't always going to be perfect and we have to be able to adapt when needed. Well, sometimes it can be hard to adapt or hard to not get down on ourselves if we don't have data that we can look back on to have things make sense. And this is where doing something like keeping track of your mood and energy levels makes so much sense. You'll be able to look back and see that you weren't feeling too good on a certain day and that's what caused you to eat more than you usually do. Here are some of the benefits you'll experience by tracking these things:

You'll Notice Patterns

One of the main reasons for doing this is that you'll start to notice patterns. For instance, you might notice that when your energy levels are below average, you tend to eat more. You might notice that for some reason you eat more on Wednesdays but you're never sure why. You now have something you can look to to help you start searching for answers. Keeping a log of these things may sound trivial, and that's why most people never think to do it. I want you to think about this though. Have you ever written something down in vague terms or shorthand, and told yourself you'd understand what you meant when you looked back at it later? However, when you looked back at the note you wrote down, you can't remember what it was you were referring to? I know this has happened to me plenty of times, which is why I always write my notes in as much detail as possible. I want the me a year from now to be able to read that note and know exactly what I was referring to. The same type of thing can happen with your nutrition. If you're looking back at a food log from a few weeks or months ago, you might be puzzled as to what was going on that day that caused you to eat more than you usually do. When you track your mood and energy levels like I'm about to describe to you, you'll know the reasoning. This is really important because when you step on the scale and the number you're hoping to see doesn't pop up, it makes you feel sad. Most people don't track anything, so they don't know the basis behind the number that they're seeing. If you know the calories you're eating and you know your feelings, then all of a sudden the number the scale is showing you will make a lot more sense.

You Can Do Something About It

Awareness is power. If you're not aware that something is a problem, how are you supposed to be able to fix it? You obviously can't, and so the first step is being aware of what your mood and energy levels are. As you start to track these things, you may notice that you're consistently low on energy. If this is true, then you're at least aware of it. Now you have the power to be able to do something about it. Maybe you can consult with a doctor, check how much sleep you're getting each and every night, and look at other things that could be causing stress in your life. Most people just try to get through the day and they never realize that their energy levels are low because they've just become so accustomed to it. That won't be the case with you luckily, and this will allow you to start to implement more habits that can help to improve these things.

How Do You Track Your Mood and Energy Levels?

Tracking your mood and energy levels doesn't have to be a complicated thing. You can use a simple spreadsheet to start to keep up with these things. All you need to do is have the date on the far left-hand column. Then in the column next to the date on the top row, you can write energy levels. In this column, you can rate your overall energy levels for the day from 1-10. In the next column over, you can label it Mood, and in this column, you'll just want to describe your overall mood for the day. What emotion or emotions would best describe your day? It could be something like normal, average, or just fine. It could be something like sad, happy, or stressful to represent a day that's above or below average. It could even be something like the first part of the day was stressful, and the second half got better. Take the day I had just yesterday as I'm writing this. My car wouldn't go above 30 mph. The dealership that's closest to my home, was booked solid for the next week. So I had to go to the next closest dealership, which was 40 minutes away. There I am taking all these different roads avoiding the main highway because I can only go 30 miles per hour. It took me forever to get there. Once I arrived, they told me they're busier than usual and it was going to need to be in the shop for 5 days. So I book a rental car online. Once I arrived, I'm told there was no rental car because their online system wasn't that good. I go to another place and get my rental car. Now I'm driving home and I start to get nauseous, I pull over and puke instantly as soon as I get out of the car. I finally got home and I'm just laying in bed in pure agony. I can't even do so much as suck on an ice cube without it making me nauseous and causing me to throw up. Later that day, I got a call saying that my engine needs to be replaced. And so yeah, that was a rough day to say the least. Luckily not all days are going to be as tough or terrible as the one I had yesterday, sometimes only part of the day is hard. This is why you can describe parts of your days if you feel that is appropriate. Sometimes though if the first part of your day is tough, it can ruin the rest of the day. The last thing you'll want to include on this sheet is a note section. This way you can recall what happened that made you feel the way you did or help you know why you might have had low energy levels on a certain day. For instance, in your notes section, you could write that you went to bed at midnight the night before. This would help to explain why your energy levels are lower than they usually are. In the notes section, you could write, car breakdown, rental car issue, excessive nausea, and throwing up. Now you'll remember that day and it will help to explain why it was so stressful. If you just write stressful and don't accompany any notes with it, it will just seem arbitrary. Yes, you'll know that you had a stressful day, but you won't know why. You won't know if something happened that was completely out of your control that you couldn't fix no matter what, or if it was something that you could work on so that way it could help to manage your emotions better. For example, with my car situation and being sick, there's nothing I could have done to manage the situation better. It was just one of those life happens situations and I just had to deal with it. Therefore, it's reasonable if my calories were off and this explanation will help to explain that. On the other hand, there are some days when I'm just angry and it's because the house is dirty. My spouse isn't picking up after himself in the kitchen. And it's not like these are unusual things. This is how it usually is in my household. But for whatever reason, some days it just gets to me more than others. By logging this in the note section, you'll be able to better see patterns and it can help you learn for the future. What was it on this day that caused me to freak out about the house being dirty when I usually don't? Maybe I had a stressful day at work and now I'm coming home and fuming on the inside. Now I need to take a second to pause and take some deep breaths to realize and understand that everything is going to be okay. For you, when there's some way that you're feeling that you are in control of, try out some different things and see what helps to regulate you the best. For me, something that helps me to calm down is taking in deep breaths. I'll inhale for 4 seconds, hold for 4 seconds, and then exhale for 4 seconds. I'll then repeat that sequence 5 times and I've found that this really helps me to be able to regulate myself. Something else that I like to do is put things in perspective. Yes, having a messy house isn't ideal, but I just think about my family and how we're all alive and okay and that's what matters most. When I start to think like that, it helps to keep me grounded. For you, it might be other things. Maybe you need to go and get regular massages to help you stay regulated. Regular massages aren't exactly cheap, so if you need an alternative, you can buy a massage gun and use that on a regular basis. Maybe you need some time to yourself where you can just veg out, watch some TV, and not have to think about things. If you're not sure what can help you decompress, just start out by trying some different things and seeing what ends up working best for you. Learning how to manage our emotions is important for our success. Too many times I've wasted hours and energy just sitting there being mad over the way things are. It doesn't matter whether it's something in my home life or with previous jobs I've had, I always look back at those moments and think to myself, "Wow, that was such a waste of time and energy." Maybe you look back at similar moments you've had in the past. And you can best believe that these moments will absolutely knock us off the fitness wagon. Instead though, if we're able to regulate our emotions, then we'll have a much easier time being able to stay the course.

Chapter 6: Low-Frequency, High-Volume Workout Routine

Yes, the primary focus of this book is to get the biggest bang for your calorie buck when it comes to nutrition. Regardless, it wouldn't be wise to only talk about nutrition and not talk about exercise. Exercise combined with nutrition can help to create an unstoppable force that will make you unstoppable for reaching your goals. The thing is, you might not like the idea of exercising. I know that it can seem like a drag to a lot of people. Let's face the facts here though. Having to eat less calories and eat healthy isn't fun all of the time either. You're reading this book for a reason and it's because you want to improve your health and overall fitness in an efficient manner that doesn't feel like dieting. Well, the same can be said for exercise. It's not always going to be glamorous. You're not always going to feel like doing it, but the reward you get for doing it will far outweigh any feelings you have towards it. When it comes to our diet, the name of the game is to get the most volume from the least amount of calories. Who's to say that we can't play a similar game when it comes to our workout routine? Why can't we have a low-frequency routine, but despite that low frequency, have our workout still yield just as good if not better results than most people? Most people are wasting their time with their dieting approach and the same applies to most people and their workout routines. If we're more efficient with our time and you're still able to get good results, then why wouldn't you want to lower your frequency? First, though, it's important to understand some workout parameters so that it will make more sense when I'm talking about things like frequency.

What is Workout Frequency, Volume, and Intensity?

When it comes to working out, there are a few variables that you have to think about. These are true regardless of what type of exercise routine that you're doing. The first is going to be workout frequency. This is going to be how often you're working out. For example, if you workout on Mondays, Wednesdays, and Fridays, then your workout frequency is 3 times per week. Someone who exercises Monday-Friday has a frequency of 5 times per week. Volume is the overall amount that you're doing during each workout. To use resistance training as an example, one person might do 10 exercises during each workout. Another person might only do 6 exercises. Within each exercise, there are sets and reps, but for the sake of the example, let's assume sets and reps are equal for all exercises for both people. In this case, the person doing 10 exercises per workout has a higher workout volume compared to the person only doing 6 exercises. Lastly, we have intensity. As you can imagine, this is how hard you're working out. In running, this is fairly simple as a sprint is a more intense form of running than jogging or walking. In weight lifting, this can vary due to many factors, but the main thing to describe intensity in my opinion would be pushing yourself to failure. Two people could both be doing squats. It could be a grueling exercise for one and a walk in the park for the other. Why is this the case? The first person is using a heavy enough weight that's challenging for them to lift, whereas the second person could only be lifting at 50% of their max capacity. There are also other factors such as rest periods that factor into how intense an exercise is. If you only rest for 30 seconds after a heavy set of squats, you best believe that next set is going to be far more challenging than someone who's resting 3 minutes in between sets. The point is that all of these factors intermix together to form your overall workload. Ideally, you would be able to max out frequency, volume, and intensity. As we all know though, we are humans and we have limits. We need to be able to recover from our workouts so that we can come back stronger for the next workout. And this brings up a good point, ultimately everyone has a different work capacity. Someone could be in better shape than someone else, which allows them to operate at a higher overall workload than someone else. However, no matter how good of shape you're in, you can eventually reach a point where you are overtraining. This is when you've broken down your body and it's unable to recover because you continue to break it down further, and it has yet to be able to adapt to your current workload that you're placing it under. This is why professional athletes must pay extreme attention to their routine. They need to train enough to improve, but they must also focus on their recovery to ensure that they don't overtrain.

So What's the Optimal Blend of Volume, Frequency, and Intensity?

As I stated in the previous section, you can't max out each of these three variables. In fact, a trade-off will often occur between them. For example, the higher your volume is, the lower your intensity will be. Imagine if you do one 40-yard sprint vs twenty 40-yard sprints. If you're doing 20, yes the volume is higher, but there's no way the 20th sprint is going to be as fast as the first few. The same thing applies with working out. If you do 10 sets of squats, you're not going to be able to lift as heavy of a weight on the 10th as you would on the first, assuming you're using a weight that challenges you in the first place. If the frequency is higher, then the overall volume of each workout should be lower. If it's not, then once again you're sacrificing intensity and potentially risking overtraining if frequency and volume are too high. Whether we want to admit it or not, there is a give and take when it comes to our workout routine. We simply can't have it all. This isn't the end of the world though. By deliberately choosing which factor we want to be lower, we can then put more of our attention into the other two variables. Most people don't even know about these variables in the first place, which means they can't optimize things, but we can. As you can probably guess from the totals of this chapter, we are going to willingly choose to lower our frequency. This will allow us to focus more on our volume and intensity when we do workout. And I do believe there are multiple benefits to choosing a lower-frequency workout routine.

Why Lower Frequency Makes Sense When It Comes to Working Out

When it comes to lowering workout frequency, what I'm referring to here is working out a lesser number of times. What would be considered a lower frequency vs a higher frequency? Something like 5 or 6 times per week would be on the higher side of things. Something like 2-3 times per week is going to be the sweet spot where we want to reside. It will be too hard to get much out of working out once per week, and you'd at least need to workout twice per week to help make it worthwhile. Why is it then that we can get more out of 2-3 workouts per week as opposed to 5-6? Well, don't even think about it from a fitness perspective. Instead, think about it through the lens of your schedule. My guess is that you're a busy person and each workout that you do is automatically going to eat up time outside of the workout itself. It doesn't matter if you're working out at home or a commercial gym, you still have to shower afterward and that's not even to mention the drive time if you are working out at a commercial gym. And this is why a lower frequency can help out tremendously. Think about the person who works out 6 times per week as opposed to the person who works out 3 times per week. Each person drives to a gym that's 10 minutes away from their home. The first person is going to spend 120 minutes or two hours just driving to the gym and back. The second person is only going to spend one hour. Right off the bat, that's an extra hour saved, and the only variable we're tweaking is frequency. It might feel like we're worse off, but this is not the case if everything else is on point.

Is it better to work 4 10s or 5 8s?

Think about it from a work perspective. Would you rather go to work 4 times per week or 5? The overall hours are the same, but the difference is you're spending more time getting ready, driving to work, getting stuck in traffic, etc. when you're working 5 days. Not only that but when you work 4 10s, you're getting off at a time when the traffic should be lessened, which helps you save even more time. Either that or you're going in earlier than most, which means you get to avoid the morning traffic. And the overall work volume is the same. Even if you don't like the idea of this in your professional life, it's the same concept that can be applied to your workout routine and it works out great. Sure in your profession, you might be needed 5 days a week anyways, so it wouldn't work that well for you to switch to a 4 day 10 hour work week. For working out though, the downside is essentially nonexistent so long as we're smart with our volume and intensity.

Most People Don't Have Time

One of the most common reasons people give for why they don't workout is because they don't have the time. And with the busy lives that most of us are living, this makes a lot of sense. Here's a look at my current schedule: wake up early and write this book, feed my son and get him ready for daycare, go to work, come home and be with family, cook, get my son ready for bed, cleaning and dishes, workout, time to get ready for bed. Most days

I'm not able to start my workout until 8:30 or 9 p.m., and that's just the way life is with a one-year-old. When I have days off from working out, I cherish them so much because it gives me personal time to do what I want once my son goes to sleep. And this is why I want to minimize the frequency as much as I can. If you have a full-time job and kids, then I'm sure your schedule looks similar to mine. Yes, I do have the time to workout, but sometimes I just don't feel like it. By working out less times during the week, dealing with this feeling becomes less of an issue.

You Can Experience Other Benefits as Well

The other thing I like about a lower-frequency workout routine is that it can help with recovery. Even if you split up your muscles to where you're working out your push muscles one day and then your pull muscles the next, your body as a unit is not getting a break. Your joints and nervous system are not getting a break. When you're only working out 2-3 times per week, there's always going to be at least one day of rest in between your workouts. This gives your full body a chance to rest and prepare for the next workout. If you're young and or a beginner, you might not notice the difference too much on your recovery. For me though, I certainly notice a difference when I'm able to take a rest day in between workouts, and that simply isn't possible when you're working out many times throughout the week.

What Does a Low-Frequency Workout Routine Look Like?

The key to pulling off a low-frequency workout routine is to ensure that the volume and intensity are on point. This is true if it's cardio or if it's in regards to lifting weights. And this brings up a good point, should you do cardio, resistance training, or both? Well, that's totally up to you. Some people feel more comfortable with cardio and don't like the idea of resistance training. Other people only want to do resistance training and don't like cardio so much. And you can of course get the best of both worlds by doing both. Do keep in mind though that lifting weights doesn't have to involve smashing some heavy weights at a commercial gym. I totally understand if the idea of that sounds uncomfortable to you. Resistance training just means that you're training your body under resistance. This resistance could even be your own body weight or it could be something like a set of resistance bands in the comfort of your own home. Either way, the first thing you need to decide is which one you want to do or if you want to do both. What won't be changing is the frequency. You'll need to decide if you want to exercise 2 or 3 times per week, and your decision will be based on what type of exercise you're going to be doing. For instance, let's say you want to focus on both cardio and resistance training. In this case, I recommend one of the following options:

-Resistance Training Twice per week and cardio once per week

-Resistance training and cardio twice per week during the same workout

-Resistance training and cardio three times per week during the same workout

If you're new to exercising or haven't done it much in recent times, then you'll want to start with a light workload and build your way up. This might mean only one resistance training workout and one cardio workout per week. You can eventually build your way up to something more than this. The ideal scenario though is that you do at least two resistance training workouts per week as that's what's necessary to maintain muscle mass (9). Which main option you choose will depend on how much time you have. If you want to save time, then splitting up your weight and cardio sessions is a good idea. However, this will limit the frequency of your cardio routine. You can stack them and do both during the same workout, but it will take a bit more time. If you're doing just cardio or resistance training, then the realm of possibilities are a lot simpler. You can do cardio or weight training 2 or 3 times per week. The same principles applies here, if you haven't exercised in months or years, then start light and build momentum. In this case that's going to be 2 times per week and then you can implement 3 times per week if you feel up to it. If you notice that you're unable to maintain 3 times per week, you can always bump things back down to 2 times per week. If in the beginning, you notice that you're struggling to consistently exercise even 2 times per week, don't sweat it. Lower the volume or frequency to a point that you feel you're able to maintain. This may only mean one workout per week. It may mean cutting your workouts down to 10 minutes apiece. You have to start with where you're at. The problem most people face is more of a mental one. You think you have to workout for an hour for it to be worthwhile. Then when it comes time to workout, it's too much for you to do so you skip. You would've had time for 10 minutes, but you didn't think you'd get anything out of it, so you ended up doing nothing. It's important to drop that mentality and instead adopt the mentality that something is better than nothing. Tell yourself that over and over again until you feel comfortable doing shorter workouts. The shorter workouts will allow you to build momentum and increase the volume of each workout you do until you reach a point of exercising for up to 45 minutes, which is all that you really need.

What Would a Low-Frequency Resistance Training Workout Look Like?

Considering the fact that you're only working out at most 3 times per week, you have to be efficient with the time you do have in the gym. Doing a typical bodybuilder split where you focus on one muscle per workout isn't going to work. That split works better if you're exercising at a frequency of at least 5 times per week. Instead, a total body workout is going to be your best friend. This is true regardless if you're doing resistance training 1, 2, or 3 times per week. As long as you have at least one day of rest in between workouts then you're good to go. Why is this so effective? Remember what I talked about earlier with working out at least twice per week to maintain muscle mass? Well, that's true if you're hitting each muscle at least two times over the course of the week. Since you're working out each muscle during your workout, you'll achieve this even if you're working out only two times per week. This is how you keep frequency low and maximize efficiency. The trade-off is that each workout will naturally be a little bit longer because we do have a lot that has to be covered. Make no mistake though, we will be efficient with the exercises that we do. And let's say you only have 10 minutes and not 45 to complete the entire workout, what do you do in those instances? Just take things from the top and complete the first couple of exercises. Then pick up where you left off for the next workout. So if you did exercises one and two during your first workout, during your next workout, you would do exercises 3 and 4. Simple as that! Here's the workout itself:

-Squats with bodyweight, band, or dumbbell
3x12
-Dumbbell Floor Press, Resistance Band
Pushups, or Bodyweight Pushups 3x12
-Seated Band Row or One Arm dumbbell Row
3x12
-Overhead tricep extensions with band or
dumbbell 3x12
-Standing Curls with band or dumbbell 3x12
-Front raises with band or dumbbell 3x12
-Bicycle Crunch 3x20

There you have it! This is an extremely simple, yet effective workout routine that you can do. You may have noticed that each exercise you see something like 3x12. What this means is you're doing 3 sets and 12 reps of the exercise. You'd do the exercise 12 times, take a rest, do it another 12 times, take a rest, and then finally do another 12 times before moving onto the next exercise. In between each set, you can take 60 seconds of rest but this can be adjusted based on your current fitness level.

What type of Cardio Routine Should I Do?

When it comes to cardio we want to be as efficient as we can be. The best way to go about that is going to be with high-intensity cardio. The downside to high intensity is that you'll fatigue sooner and you can only do it for so long. This is why we want to alternate it with low-intensity cardio, such as walking. For this workout, this means you would go as fast as you can for as long as you can. Then once you fatigue, you would walk for as long as you need and then you would repeat the cycle. You can do this for varying amounts of time. If you're doing this after a weight training workout, then you can do it for a shorter period of time, such as 10-15 minutes. If you're doing a workout that's just cardio then you can do it for 20-30 minutes. Just like with resistance training, you can build your way up. If 20-30 minutes is too hard for you, then start with 5-10 minutes. If going at a high intensity is too much for you, then try a light jog or even walking for the entire duration. Remember something is better than nothing, so don't feel like walking is a waste because it's not!

Conclusion

Dieting does not have to be as hard as people make it out to be. As long as you're smart with the calories you do have to eat, then it will hardly feel as if you're dieting at all. The problem for most people is they're either too restrictive or they push the envelope and eat too much junk food. Either of these things puts people in a bind. You won't have to worry about either of these problems though. You'll be able to feel full and still lose weight. You'll also get to enjoy some of your favorite foods from time to time. You'll get to have your cake and eat it too, which is sadly something that most will never figure out how to do when it comes to their health and nutrition.

Sources

(1) https://www.medicalnewstoday.com/articles/is-it-better-to-eat-several-small-meals-or-fewer-larger-ones#Meal-frequency-and-weight-loss

(2) https://www.ncbi.nlm.nih.gov/pmc/articles/PMC9967803/

(3) https://pubmed.ncbi.nlm.nih.gov/17848938/#:~:text=Abstract,32.2%20MJ%20kg(%2D1).

(4) https://pubmed.ncbi.nlm.nih.gov/34833893/

(5) https://pubmed.ncbi.nlm.nih.gov/36059207/

(6) https://pubmed.ncbi.nlm.nih.gov/31336535/

(7) https://www.ncbi.nlm.nih.gov/pmc/articles/PMC6209729/

(8) https://pubmed.ncbi.nlm.nih.gov/31082163/

(9) https://pubmed.ncbi.nlm.nih.gov/33629972/#:~:text=Strength%20and%20muscle%20size%20(at,for%20athletes%20or%20military%20personnel.